boost
energy

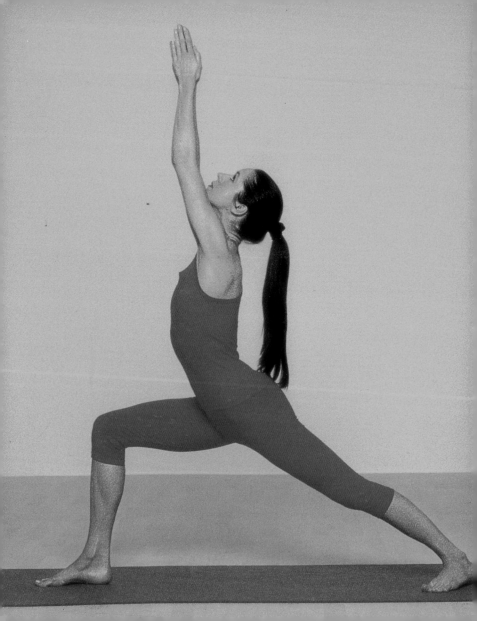

boost
energy

Peter Falloon-Goodhew

YOGA BIOMEDICAL TRUST

DK Publishing

London, New York, Munich,
Melbourne, and Delhi

Series art editor: Anne-Marie Bulat
Series editor: Jane Laing
Series consultant: Peter Falloon-Goodhew
Managing editor: Gillian Roberts
Senior art editor: Karen Sawyer
Category publisher: Mary-Clare Jerram
US editor: Maggi McCormick
DTP designer: Sonia Charbonnier
Production controller: Joanna Bull

Photographer: Graham Atkins-Hughes
(represented by A & R Associates)

First American Edition, 2002

02 03 04 05 10 9 8 7 6 5 4 3 2 1

Published in the United States by
DK Publishing, Inc.
375 Hudson Street
New York, New York 10014

ISBN: 0-7894-8905-8

Color reproduced in Singapore by
Colourscan
Printed and bound in Hong Kong / China by
South China Printing Co.

See our complete product line at
www.dk.com

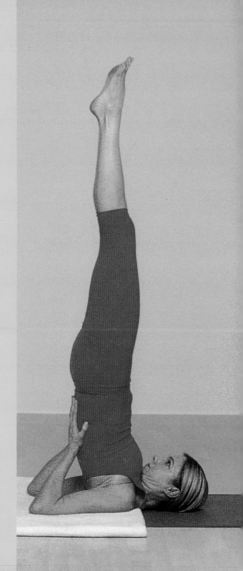

contents

introduction

The appeal of yoga is universal and timeless. Its holistic practices work on the physical, mental, emotional, and spiritual planes, boosting your energy levels and helping you live more positively.

Yoga is a tried-and-tested practical method of achieving all-around good health. It does not seek to offer a quick fix, but provides a long-term program for living positively. Its combination of physical postures, breathing practices, relaxation, meditation, and lifestyle guidance can help you stay physically fit and mentally alert, and live more positively and mindfully. For many people, yoga becomes a lifelong journey of self-discovery, bringing peace of mind and inner happiness.

Unlike some forms of exercise, yoga is suitable for everyone. Whatever your age or level of fitness, yoga is a very safe form of exercise, provided you work within your limits. However, please read through the text in the box below, entitled "Health Concerns," before you begin, since some yoga practices can be physically demanding.

HEALTH CONCERNS

If a health practitioner has advised you not to overexert yourself physically, or if you have any other health concerns, seek advice from a qualified yoga therapist or teacher (see p.128) before using this book. Page 17 provides basic advice for some common medical conditions and, where appropriate, "Take Care" advice or Alternatives are given for individual practices. If you are pregnant, or have recently given birth, ask a suitably qualified yoga teacher which practices would be appropriate for you.

Life is energy

Human beings are complex energy systems, with energy processes taking place at physical, mental, emotional, and spiritual levels. The simplest form of energy is metabolic. This derives from the food we eat and the air we breathe. There is also vital energy – feeling glad to be alive and bursting with health.

For many people, vital energy is no more than an expression of the collective physical energies generated by the way mind and body work together. But for others it is the secret ingredient that makes the difference. In yoga, this vital energy is known as *prana*, the embodiment of the universal life force that flows everywhere and through everything – the "intelligence" behind creation.

Symptoms of low energy

Whatever you believe, everyone accepts that feeling good does not depend simply on how much energy you possess, but also on whether it is flowing freely. Sometimes energy becomes blocked, resulting in low levels of energy or an imbalance

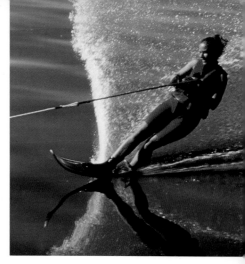

High energy levels give you a zest for life that makes you physically active, positive-thinking, and emotionally robust.

between physical, mental, and emotional energies.

If you are suffering from low levels of energy, you may find that, while you can cope with your normal day-to-day routine, anything that requires a little more effort tires you quickly. You may lack strength or stamina. Or you may have a general feeling of being physically "out of sorts" in which you wake up feeling tired.

Reduced energy levels may be expressed in poor postural habits and a lack of spring in your step. You may find that you are more susceptible to colds and other minor ailments. In extreme cases, you may find that virtually everything you do tires you or leaves you feeling weak.

Mentally, you may find that your concentration levels are so low that you find it difficult to keep your mind on your work, or to read a book or watch television without becoming distracted or bored. Remembering things and making decisions may be more difficult. You may find it difficult to raise much enthusiasm for doing anything at all.

At an emotional level, symptoms of low energy include becoming more easily irritated and upset and more susceptible to anger, fear, jealousy, or envy. You may find yourself more critical of the world, your family, and your friends, and find it harder to accept change. As such negative emotions take hold, you become less able to laugh and to participate in and enjoy life. You become easily dragged down by events, tending to see problems rather than opportunities in new situations. Such feelings themselves drain you of energy.

Causes of low energy
The causes of low or out-of-balance energy levels are many and varied. There may be a single, identifiable cause, but more often there will be several factors contributing to your lack of energy, including:
• underlying medical conditions
• unbalanced diet
• sedentary lifestyle
• sleep deprivation
• stressful life situations.

Underlying medical conditions
Low energy levels may indicate an underlying medical problem. Conditions commonly associated with fatigue include depression, anxiety, and insomnia. Recovering from viral illnesses, anemia, low thyroid gland function, breathing problems such as severe asthma and hyperventilation, uncontrolled diabetes, and chronic pain (for example, back pain or arthritis) can also cause fatigue.

Prolonged fatigue may also be associated with more serious illnesses, so consult your doctor if you are worried.

Unbalanced diet

A well-balanced diet is essential to high energy levels. Nutritional inputs must keep pace with the demands of metabolism, and both undereating and overeating can adversely affect energy levels. So can eating over-processed food, and foods that contain many artificial additives and/or salt, sugar, or added flavorings. Consuming excessive quantities of foods that are potentially addictive, such as those containing caffeine and alcohol, also leads to energy imbalances.

Sedentary lifestyle

Anyone who has been incapacitated in some way for any length of time will know how quickly muscle mass and stamina can deteriorate through lack of activity. However, it does not necessarily take an accident or illness to reduce your strength and stamina.

A sedentary lifestyle, often accompanied by poor postural habits, can adversely affect digestive processes, reduce respiratory capacity, place increased strain on the cardiovascular system, and cause

YOGA AND EATING

Yoga encourages you to eat moderately and simply, to eat natural, fresh foods as far as possible, and to pay attention to how you eat. The guidelines below will help you become more aware of your eating habits. They will also help you digest food more effectively.

- Eat freshly prepared meals.
- Do not eat until the last meal has been digested (up to three hours).
- Avoid distractions while eating, such as reading the newspaper or watching television.
- Do not eat when you are angry or upset about something.
- Take small mouthfuls and chew well.
- Do not drink large amounts of water (or other fluids) during meals.
- Drink plenty of water at other times.

muscle imbalances and weakness. In addition, inactivity can cause mental dullness, leading to a vicious circle of mental and physical fatigue.

Sleep deprivation

Sleep deprivation is a common problem (eight hours' sleep is about the right amount for most people). Unless a sleep debt is made up in the following days, the debt grows. So, while you may superficially become used to an inadequate sleep regime, your immune system and the body's repair and "battery recharging" mechanisms suffer. This can result in poor reaction times, concentration, memory, and physical performance, and in poor judgment and frequent mood swings.

Our body rhythms can be upset by lifestyles that deviate strongly from the powerful sleep-regulating stimuli of sunrise and nightfall. Shift workers are often affected, feeling drowsy at work and unable to sleep when they get home. At worst, digestive, cardiovascular, emotional, and mental problems may result.

Stressful life situations

Long hours spent at your workplace or heavy workloads, particularly if the work involves repetitive or boring tasks, can be draining both mentally and physically.

Bringing up a young family can be challenging, and combining it with a busy job inevitably adds to the pressures. Many people are

continually working against the clock, trying to fit in as many tasks as possible. This can sap energy and result in a dependency on stimulants, such as nicotine, to help get through the day, and on alcohol to wind down at the end of it. The benefits of these substances are fleeting and the adverse effects long-term.

In addition, financial worries, strained relationships, feeling lonely, and other personal problems can all reduce energy reserves, fostering a negative approach to life in general.

How yoga can help

The central purpose of yoga is to enable us to experience the limitless life energy that is the core of our being. Normally this is impossible because we are too enmeshed in the web of our daily lives. We tend to be too preoccupied with our desires, our attachment to objects and people, our prejudices and dislikes, and with the physical, mental, and emotional stresses that flow from them.

The way to overcome this limited way of living is to be able to "let go." Patanjali, a great yoga sage who lived over 2,000 years ago, described it as being able to "still the thought waves of the mind." Bringing the mind to a state of quiet calm is not easy, but it can be done by practicing the physical postures, breathing practices, relaxation, concentration, and meditation that together comprise the practice of yoga.

Practicing the physical postures brings improvements in cardiovascular endurance, muscle strength, flexibility, balance and coordination, and body reaction times. Gradually, your self-esteem and your life energy improve. Simply by regularly practicing the postures, you become generally more alive both physically and mentally.

Patanjali taught that we must change the habitual ways we think and act. He offered guidance on how we should relate to other people and to the world around us with a set of

MAXIMS FOR LIVING

A positive relationship with the world and with yourself was of fundamental importance to Patanjali. Try to live by his maxims (interpreted below). They will help you live more positively, allowing life energy to flow more freely through you.

In your relationship with the world around you, you should:

• Avoid causing harm; endeavor to be compassionate.
• Be honest in all your thoughts, words, and actions.
• Never steal from others. This applies not only to possessions, but also to wasting other people's time, energy, and goodwill.
• Be faithful and selfless in all your personal relationships.
• Avoid acquiring or holding on to material things (or people) for the sake of it, or for selfish reasons.

In relation to yourself, you should work to:

• Develop purity in mind, body, and spirit – inner and outer cleanliness.
• Pursue simplicity in life, and try to make the most of whatever life brings.
• Develop physical and mental resolve (through yoga practices) to withstand difficulties and disappointments in life.
• Learn to identify with your inner self rather than with your habitual ways of acting and seeing situations.
• Accept that there is more to life than the material world, and be respectful of the intelligence underpinning life.

personal observances designed to encourage a healthy, positive approach to life. In essence, he taught mindfulness: "being with what is." This means giving all of your attention to whomever you are with or whatever you are doing, and not allowing yourself to be carried away by some distracting train of thought or letting your emotions cloud your sense of judgment.

New approach to life

Because most of us are used to living in ways that put our egos, our desires and attachments, our prejudices, and our hopes and fears at the center, letting go and acting in a selfless manner is difficult. And it is not just a question of the actions themselves, but the spirit in which they are done; we need to enjoy our selfless actions, not do them grudgingly.

If you are able to let go of negative attitudes and emotions, rather than giving way to them or suppressing them; if you respect others, show compassion, and learn to follow your heart, then you will find that your energy levels naturally rise. And you will become less susceptible to being worn down by the negativity of others. These are not changes that can be achieved overnight. You must work at them consistently, trying to be more objective and more discriminating, and to consciously cultivate positive attitudes.

Take one of Patanjali's principles of behavior and attitude (see "Maxims for Living," p.11), and

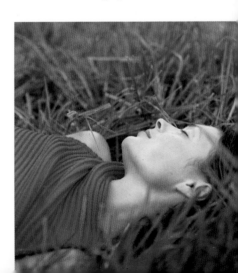

Go for a walk in the country or by the sea and reflect on your attitudes and behavior toward others. Meditate on the beauty and the stillness of nature.

observe how close you get to it in your thoughts, intentions, and actions during the course of a day. The next day, make a positive effort to behave in accordance with the same principle, and observe the difference in the way you feel when you do. Work your way through all the maxims in this fashion. Provided you work with determination and are not discouraged by setbacks, you will find yourself gradually becoming more aware, more mindful, more energized – and happier!

Trying to be more in tune with nature and finding more time for yourself can help, too. Paying attention to, and appreciating, the world around you, and marveling at the wonders of nature, can be especially helpful in enabling you to appreciate the intelligence underlying the universe, and to be less self-centered. Last, if you can spend time in the countryside or open spaces, away from the activity, noise, and pollution of modern society, you can benefit energetically simply from the quietness and the improved quality of the air you breathe.

HOW TO USE THIS BOOK

The remainder of this book is divided into three sections. The **Foundations** section provides guidance on doing yoga and some basic breathing and preliminary stretches. Familiarize yourself with these first before moving on to the **Building Blocks** section. This contains a selection of postures and breathing practices, as well as a simple meditation and relaxation technique. Work through these postures gradually, selecting one or two to work on at a time, rather than trying to do them all at once. Look at the photographs first to get a feel for the overall shape of the posture. Then follow the accompanying step-by-step instructions carefully. If you find a posture difficult to do, try the alternative, if one is given.

The **Programs** section combines selected postures and other practices in a series of short yoga programs designed for particular situations and needs. Make sure that you understand how to do the postures first before trying these programs.

Yoga is traditionally learned from a teacher, and you will benefit from going to a class, if you are not already doing so. Organizations that can help you find a qualified teacher are listed on page 128.

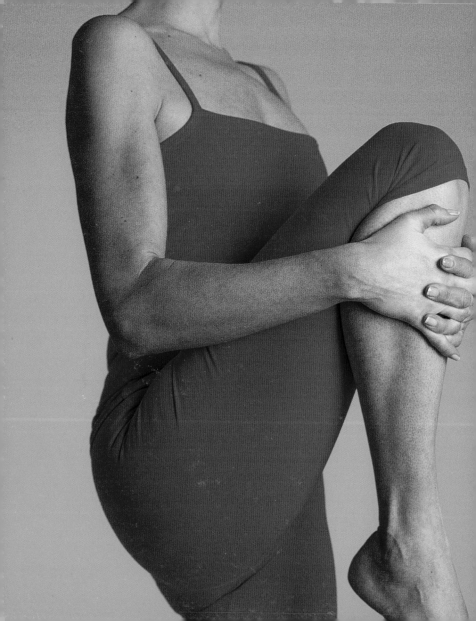

part 1

foundations

This section provides advice for those new to yoga. It includes basic standing, sitting, and lying positions; preliminary practices to bring awareness to your yoga practice, and breathe-and-stretch exercises to loosen the body and help coordinate breath with movement.

before
you start

The practice of yoga begins with your attitude. Take time to read the general guidance provided in this section. It will help make your practice meaningful and mindful.

Try to establish a regular time to practice yoga. It is better to do a little yoga every day rather than a lot once or twice a week. Before breakfast or in the early evening are good times.

Always practice on an empty stomach. Allow three hours to elapse after a large meal, two hours after a light meal, and one hour after a snack before starting your yoga practice. Wear comfortable clothes that do not restrict your movement or breathing in any way. Practice on a sticky mat or other nonslip surface and make sure you have enough space around you to extend.

If you have not done yoga before, make sure you do not overreach

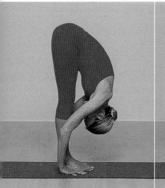
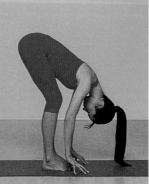

WORK WITHIN YOUR LIMITS

Never force your body into a posture. Gentler alternatives are possible for most yoga postures. Shown here are the full and the modified versions of the Forward Bend (see p.38).

yourself during your early yoga sessions. To begin with, you may feel some stiffness for one or two days afterward, but it will soon pass.

Nothing you do should cause you pain. If you do feel pain, ease off. If you feel chest pain, experience heart irregularity, feel dizzy, or become short of breath, stop immediately. If practicing more gently does not solve the problem, seek medical advice.

Never try to compete with others or with images you have seen in a book. Just as importantly, do not be competitive and impatient with yourself. Everyone has different strengths and weaknesses. Let your guiding principle be to work from within your limits, seeking to extend those limits gradually, but without exceeding them.

Always practice yoga in a balanced way. Counterpose strong, forward-bending postures with backbends, and counterpose backbends with forward-bending postures or some twists. After working one side of the body in a posture, always repeat the sequence on the other side.

YOGA AND COMMON MEDICAL CONDITIONS

• If you have high blood pressure (HBP), a heart condition, glaucoma, or a detached retina, do not let your head stay below your heart.

• If you have HBP or a heart condition, hold strong standing and prone postures for a short time only. In addition, for HBP, keep your arms below your head.

• If you have low blood pressure (LBP), come up slowly from inverted poses.

• If you have a back problem or sciatica, avoid bending and twisting movements that provoke pain or other symptoms (for example, tingling or numbness in the leg). Keep your knees bent in forward bends.

• If you have a hernia, or have had recent abdominal surgery, do not put strong pressure on the abdomen.

• If you have arthritis, mobilize joints to their maximum pain-free range, but rest them if they are inflamed.

• If you have arthritis of the neck or other neck problems, do not tilt the head back in backbends and be cautious with sideways and twisting neck movements.

• During menstruation, energy levels may be lower than usual, and you may need to practice more gently. Avoid inversions and postures that put strong pressure on the pelvic area.

the basics

In yoga, basic standing, sitting, and lying down positions are important in their own right, helping you develop stability and awareness of the benefits of alignment for your posture, your breathing, and for the free flow of energy. They also provide the foundations from which other postures are developed.

In addition, being able to sit comfortably and steadily is important for breathing practices and also for meditation, helping you remain focused without distractions from physical tensions. Lying down is often used to develop body and breath awareness, and to relax and let your body absorb the beneficial effects of other yoga practices.

If you find it impossible to achieve the full posture, it can be very helpful to use a prop, such as a block or cushion, ensure that you do not strain your body.

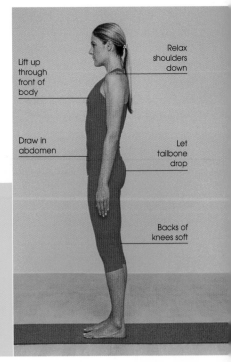

Lift up through front of body

Relax shoulders down

Draw in abdomen

Let tailbone drop

Backs of knees soft

STANDING

Stand up straight with your feet parallel, hip-width apart, and your ears, tops of shoulders, hips, and ankles in line. Press your feet to the ground and lift upward through your body. Broaden across the top of the chest. Feel yourself balanced in every direction, head as if suspended by a thread from the ceiling. Look straight ahead, relax, and breathe easily.

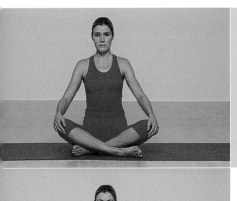

EASY SITTING

This basic posture is good for breathing practices. Cross your shins with each foot under the opposite calf or knee. Position yourself on the front edge of your sitting bones, with the spine long and the head erect. Relax the shoulders. If your knees are higher than your hips, sit on a block or another support.

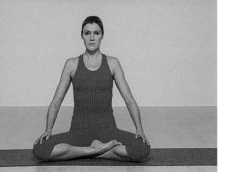

ADVANCED SITTING

If you are fairly flexible, this is a more stable position for prolonged sitting (for example, in meditation). Sit with your legs spread. Bring the sole of your left foot against the inside of your right thigh and your right foot on to, or in front of, your left calf, with the heels touching. Your knees should be resting on the floor. Do not strain to sit in the posture.

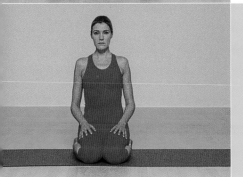

KNEELING

Try this position if you find basic cross-legged sitting uncomfortable. Sit on your heels with the tops of your thighs facing the ceiling. Alternatively, if you are going to stay longer, position your knees and feet hip-width apart and sit on blocks, a folded blanket, or a bolster. Keep your spine long and your head erect, with the shoulders and the neck relaxed.

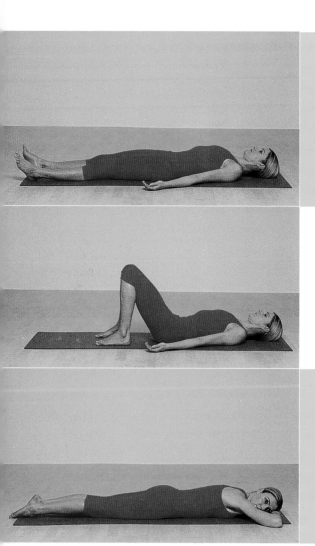

LYING ON BACK

Lie with your legs stretched out, feet hip-width apart. Allow the feet and legs to roll out. Place your arms away from the body, backs of the hands on the floor. Relax the neck and rest the center of the back of the head on the floor.

LYING WITH LEGS BENT

If you feel any discomfort in your lower back when lying flat, having your legs bent can be a good alternative. Keep your feet hip-width apart and let the knees rest against each other.

LYING ON FRONT

Between prone postures you might like to relax by lying on your front. Keep your feet hip-width apart and use the backs of your hands as a pillow on which to rest your turned head. Let the legs relax and the heels fall outward.

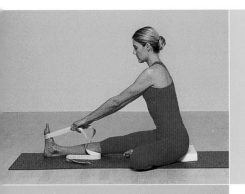

USING BELTS AND BLOCKS

Belts and blocks can be used in a wide variety of situations as supports and stabilizers to help you practice postures effectively without straining yourself. For example, in forward-bending movements – as shown here – using a belt helps protect the back if you have tight hamstrings or tight hips.

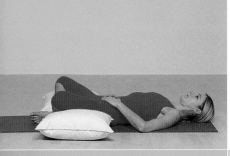

USING PILLOWS

Pillows can be used to support different parts of the body. Here they are shown supporting the thighs in Supine Butterfly (see p.92), allowing the inner and the outer thigh muscles to relax, the hips to open farther, and the person to stay in the posture longer without being distracted by discomfort.

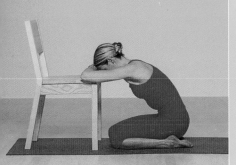

USING A CHAIR

Chairs can be used to modify postures. Shown here is a version of Child (see p.74) for someone with HBP. A chair can also be used for breathing or meditation practices if sitting or kneeling on the floor is uncomfortable. Sit toward the front of the chair, with the soles of the feet flat on the floor (or block), hands resting on the thighs or in the lap.

centering

Take a few minutes before starting your yoga practice to settle the mind and body by focusing on the here and now. This technique is known as centering, and helps develop awareness and mindfulness.

You can center yourself by standing, sitting, or lying down quietly for a few minutes in a comfortable position. Simply observe your breath, letting it settle into a quiet, natural rhythm. As you do so, the activity in your mind will lessen. However, if your body is stiff and your muscles tense, you will find the following lying down centering relaxation practice helpful before starting to do the postures.

lying down centering

1 Lie on the floor with your knees bent, feet hip-width apart. Place your arms away from the sides of the body, the backs of the hands on the floor, and the fingers gently curling inward. Position the center of the back of the head on the floor, and relax the neck. If your neck feels strained, try placing a small support (for example, a block, thin pillow, or folded blanket) underneath your head.

2 Allow your lower back to sink toward the floor. Slide your feet along the floor to stretch the legs out. Let the legs relax and the feet fall outward. (If you feel discomfort in your back, keep your knees bent.) Close your eyes. Be aware of how balanced your body feels. Are the different parts of the body sinking into the floor equally, or are there tensions or restrictions in some areas?

3 Slowly take your attention to each part of your body, starting with the feet and working upward through the lower legs, upper legs, hips, buttocks, hands, lower arms, upper arms, chest, lower back, shoulders, neck, and face. Ask each part of the body to relax and allow them all to release down into the floor. Become aware of your breath and make sure you are breathing through your nostrils. Do not try to control the breath or change it in any way; simply observe its movement in and out of the body. Let your breath settle into a slow, deep, natural rhythm. Each time you breathe out be aware of letting go. Feel the body "sinking" into the floor, while at the same time it is supported by the floor.

4 Bring your attention to your out-breath. Allow it to become a little longer than your in-breath. Now count down 10 out-breaths. The breath should remain calm and unhurried as you count. When you reach zero, gently turn the head from side to side three times. Then, on an in-breath, stretch your arms up to the ceiling and then behind you. Stretch through to the fingertips as you press your lower back to the floor and your heels gently toward the wall in front of you. Relax into the stretch for a few breaths. Then, on an out-breath, bring your arms back down to your sides, or to rest on your abdomen, and let go completely. Gently turn onto one side of your body, pause for a moment, then slowly sit or stand up.

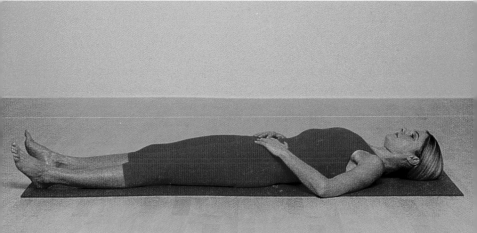

basic
breathing

There is a fundamental connection between the breath and your physical, mental, and emotional states. The breath is the pathway for *prana* – "the breath behind the breath" – to enter the body.

Breathing provides oxygen for the metabolic processes from which we derive the energy to move, think, and feel, and carries away carbon dioxide, the main waste product of metabolism. Physical tension in the respiratory muscles between and deep to the ribs can cause tightness in the chest, and even chest pain. Relaxed breathing techniques will release tension from the whole of the upper body, including the neck and shoulders. This will improve your ability to adjust your breathing to meet changing requirements.

The breath also provides a powerful link between mind and body. By controlling your breathing patterns – for example, the rhythm and depth of breathing, the length of the out-breath, and the balance between right and left nostrils – you can influence your physical, mental, and emotional states.

Good breathing habits

Yoga encourages breathing through the nose, full use of the diaphragm, a slow, smooth breathing pattern, and coordination of movement and breath. In the poses, opening movements, such as backbends, are usually done on an in-breath and closing movements, such as forward bends, on an out-breath.

The breathing practice opposite will help develop awareness of the respiratory muscles and encourage good breathing habits. It can also be done standing or lying down.

sitting sectional breathing

Sectional breathing helps unlock energy blocks associated with poor breathing habits. After completing

Step 3, combine all three steps to produce full, continuous in-breaths and out-breaths.

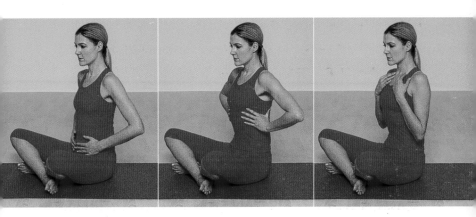

1 Sit comfortably with your palms resting on your abdomen, the middle fingers just touching. Breathe into your hands, feeling the abdomen swell out and the fingers move apart as you breathe in. Then feel the abdomen sink back as you exhale. Take six even breaths.

2 Bring your hands to your ribcage, with your fingers to the front and thumbs on the back ribs. Feel the ribs expand into the hands on the in-breath and then relax back inward as you exhale. Take six breaths, keeping the abdomen as still as possible.

3 Rest the fronts of your fingers just below your collar bones. Breathe in, feeling the top of the chest expand and the fingers and shoulders rise up toward the head. As you breathe out, feel the fingers sink back down. Take six breaths.

breathe and
stretch

The following exercises work on coordinating movement with the breath, and stretching tight muscles. Being aware of your breath as you move will allow energy to flow more freely through your body.

up and down stretch

1 Assume the basic standing position (see p.18) with your feet parallel and about hip-width apart. Looking straight ahead, take several full breaths.

2 On an in-breath, sweep your arms slowly out to the side and up above your head. Bring your palms together, fingers pointing toward the ceiling. Continue to look straight ahead.

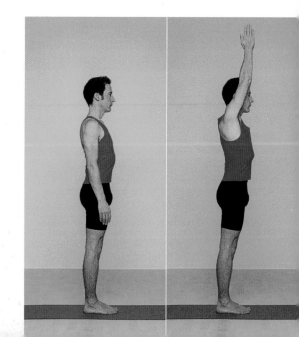

As you breathe out, fold the arms backward, bringing your palms together and hands down your back so that your fingers point toward the floor. At the same time, stretch your elbows toward the ceiling.

Interlock your fingers. As you breathe in, straighten out the arms again, stretching the palms of the hands up toward the ceiling.

Breathe out, sweeping your arms out to the sides and down. Breathe in as you take your arms back toward the wall behind you, interlocking the fingers again behind your back. Open your chest and hold in your abdomen.

Breathe out as you fold forward from the hips, with knees bent. Stretch the backs of the hands toward the ceiling. Come back up as you breathe in, stretching the arms back again. Lower the arms to the sides on the out-breath. Repeat the sequence several times.

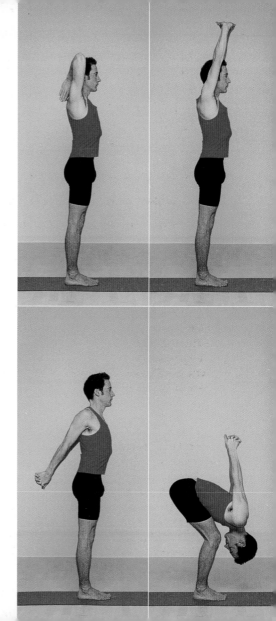

swimming breaststroke

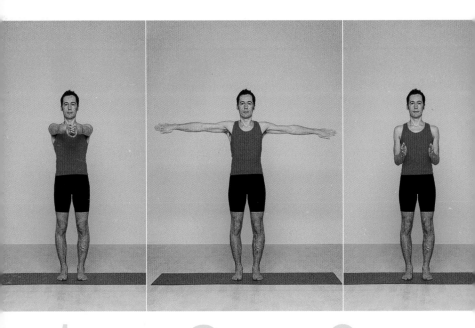

1 Stand up straight, feet parallel and hip-width apart. Stretch your arms forward at shoulder level, palms together. Take two or three breaths, then, on an in-breath, turn your palms out to bring the backs of the hands together.

2 As you breathe out, sweep the arms out to the side, then back and down to your sides in a circular motion, mimicking the arm movement of the breaststroke.

3 Keeping the elbows close to the sides of the body, stretch the arms forward and bring the palms together on the in-breath. Repeat the sequence several times, keeping the movement smooth and flowing.

swimming backstroke

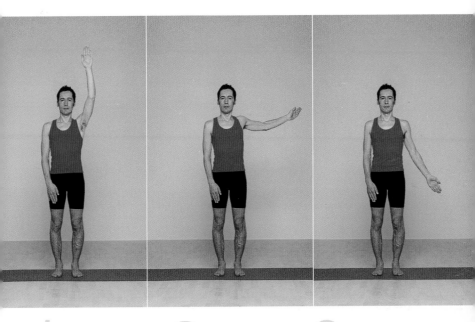

1 Stand up tall, feet parallel and hip-width apart. Place the palms of your hands on the fronts of your thighs. Let the breath settle into a regular rhythm. As you breathe in, bring your left arm forward and up toward the ceiling.

2 Continue in a circular motion, bringing your left arm behind you, as though swimming the backstroke. Press the right palm against the thigh to stop the body from twisting. Keep looking straight ahead of you.

3 Bring the arm down and forward. On the out-breath, circle the right arm back and down in the same way. Repeat several times. Then breathe in as you circle the right arm back and breathe out as you circle the left arm.

side bend and twist

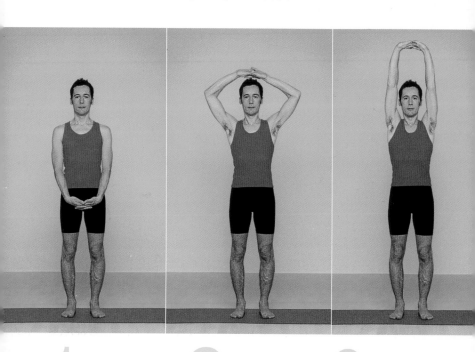

1 Assume the basic standing position, feet hip-width apart. Bring the hands together in front of the body and interlock the fingers. Take several breaths.

2 On an in-breath, roll the hands up the front of the body to bring them just above the head, with the palms facing the ceiling.

3 As you breathe out, stretch your palms toward the ceiling, keeping the shoulders down away from the ears. Lengthen through the arms.

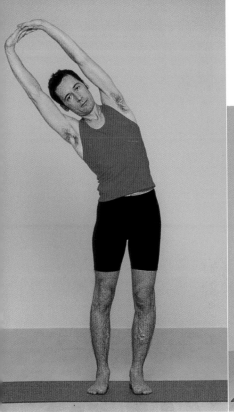

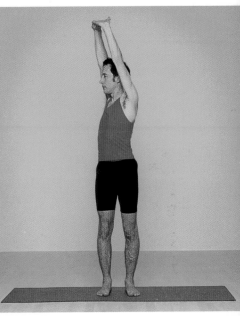

Breathe in; then, as you breathe out, bend to the right, hingeing at the waist. Breathe in as you come back up to the center. As you breathe out, bend to the left, and breathe in as you come back up again.

Breathe out as you twist to the right, keeping the palms pushing toward the ceiling. Breathe in as you come back to face the front. Breathing out, twist to the left and come back to face the front again on the in-breath. Lower your arms in front of you as you breathe out, keeping the fingers interlocked. Repeat the entire sequence twice.

one-legged stretch

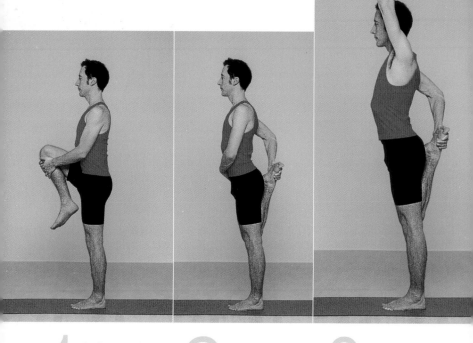

From the basic standing position, raise your right knee toward your chest and clasp your hands around the shin. Ease the knee toward the chest and take three slow, deep breaths.

Slide the right hand down to the foot and lower the knee. Press the heel against the right buttock. Place your left hand on the right hip. Take three breaths as you press the right hip forward against your left hand.

Stretch the left arm up beside the head. Take three breaths. Keeping the bent knee in line with the straight leg, release the right foot and slowly lower it to the floor. Repeat with the left leg.

knee lifts and kicks

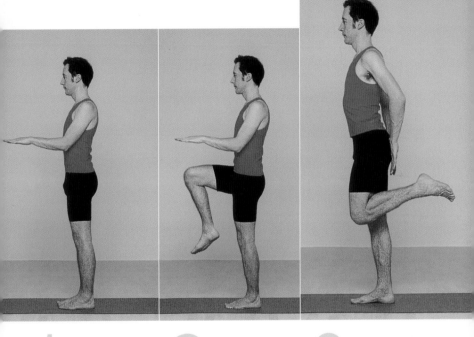

1 Assume the basic standing position, feet hip-width apart. Hold both hands out in front of you at waist level, palms facing the floor, elbows against the sides of your body. Let your breath settle into a smooth rhythm.

2 Alternately lift the right and left knee to touch the palms of the hands. Do not lower the arm or bend forward to meet the knee as it comes up. Start slowly, and gradually increase your speed.

3 Rest the backs of your hands on the buttocks. Alternately kick each leg back to touch the palm of the hand with the heel. Start slowly, gradually increasing speed. Repeat Steps 2 and 3 until slightly out of breath.

wide-legged squat

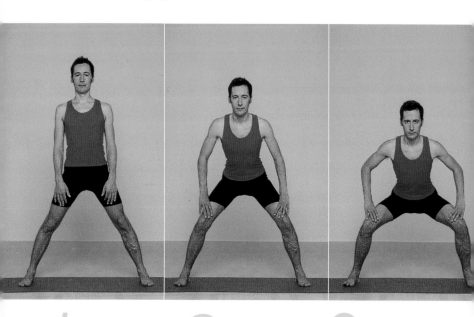

1 Stand upright with your legs about 3–4 ft (90–120 cm) apart, feet turned out a little, and knees in line with the toes. Look straight ahead.

2 Bend the knees slightly and bring your hands onto the insides of your thighs, just above your knees. Spread the fingers slightly and place the thumbs on the outside of the thighs. Take a breath in.

3 As you exhale, take your hips back as though you were going to sit down. Keep your spine long and do not let your hips sink below your knees. Come back up on the in-breath. Repeat slowly up to 10 times.

wide-legged lunge

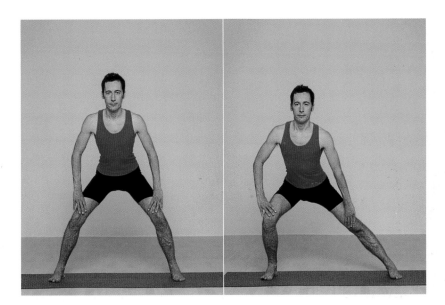

1 Stand with your knees slightly bent and your hands resting on the insides of your thighs just above the knees. Spread the fingers slightly and place the thumbs on the outside of the thighs. Take several breaths.

2 As you breathe out, lunge to the right, bending the right knee and straightening the left leg. Then lunge to the left as you breathe in. Repeat slowly up to 10 times, breathing out as you go to the left and in as you go to the right. Feel the stretch on the insides of the thighs. Make sure the bent knee stays in line with the toes.

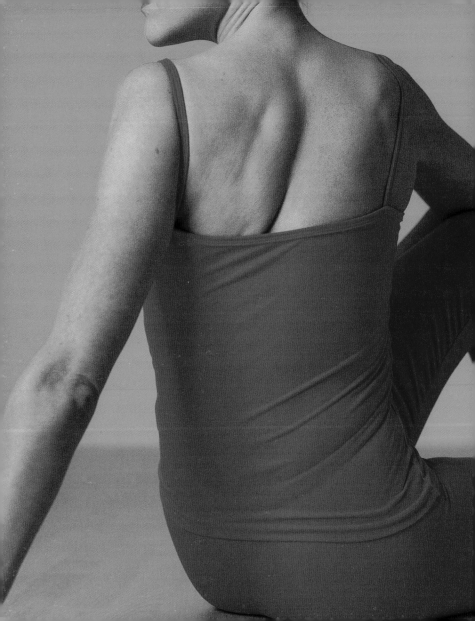

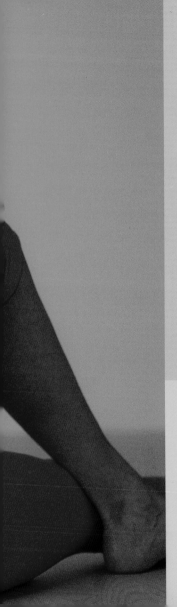

building blocks

This section presents a selection of postures and other yoga practices to revitalize your body, mind, and spirit. Stay in the postures only for as long as you are able to hold them steadily and comfortably, breathing evenly. Listen to your body as you practice and you will soon feel the benefits.

forward
bend

Take the weight off your shoulders and allow the spine to stretch with this calming posture. Keep the feet rooted and the sitting bones lifting up to help stretch tight hamstrings. Come out slowly and carefully.

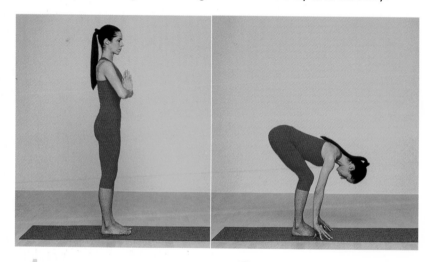

1 Assume the basic standing position (see p.18). Then bring the palms together in front of your chest in prayer position. Take several breaths, feeling yourself growing taller and becoming more relaxed.

2 As you breathe out, fold forward from the hips, bending your knees at the same time. Place your fingertips on the floor. Let the upper body rest on the thighs and keep the back long. Breathe easily.

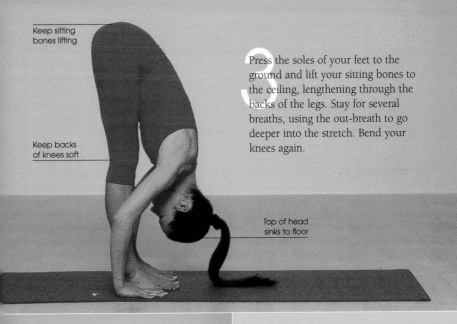

Keep sitting
bones lifting

3 Press the soles of your feet to the ground and lift your sitting bones to the ceiling, lengthening through the backs of the legs. Stay for several breaths, using the out-breath to go deeper into the stretch. Bend your knees again.

Keep backs
of knees soft

Top of head
sinks to floor

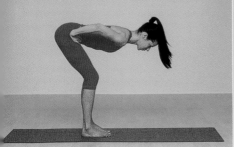

4 Put your hands on your hips and come up halfway on an in-breath. Lengthen through the spine on the out-breath. On an in-breath, hingeing from the hips and keeping your back straight, come all the way up.

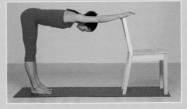

ALTERNATIVE

If you have HBP, a heart condition, glaucoma, or a detached retina, do a Half Forward Bend, resting your hands on the back or seat of a chair. Keep the abdomen gently pulled back toward the spine and the chest lifted. If you have lower back pain or sciatica, keep your knees bent.

warrior

This strong standing pose builds strength in the legs and back. Keep the tailbone dropping as you lift out of the hips toward the hands. Breathe evenly, remaining balanced and focused throughout.

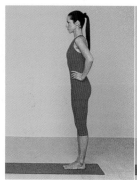 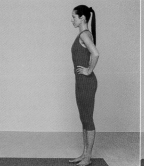 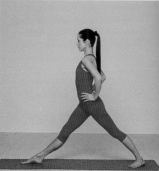

1 Stand with your feet together. Place your hands on your hips. Focus on your breath.

2 Pivoting on your heel, turn your left foot out about 45 degrees. Lift upward out of your hips as you breathe in.

3 As you exhale, take a large step forward with the right foot. Square the hips to the front, adjusting the position of your back foot if necessary. Take a breath in.

TAKE CARE
• If you have back problems, be cautious as you move into the final position. • Don't look up if you have neck problems. • If you have HBP or a heart condition, hold for a short time and keep your hands on your hips.

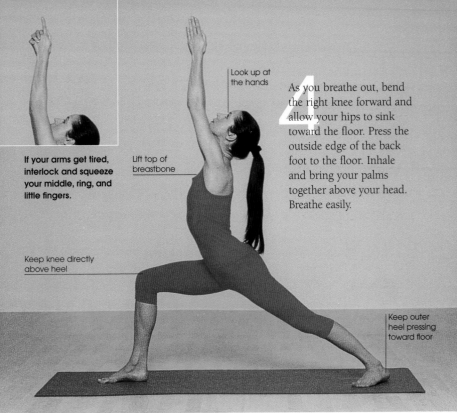

If your arms get tired, interlock and squeeze your middle, ring, and little fingers.

Look up at the hands

Lift top of breastbone

Keep knee directly above heel

Keep outer heel pressing toward floor

4 As you breathe out, bend the right knee forward and allow your hips to sink toward the floor. Press the outside edge of the back foot to the floor. Inhale and bring your palms together above your head. Breathe easily.

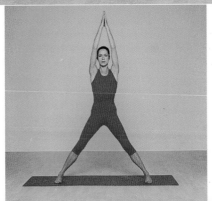

5 On an in-breath, straighten the right leg. Turn 90 degrees to come into a wide-legged position. Step your feet together and lower your arms. Repeat the sequence, turning the right foot out at Step 2 and stepping forward with the left foot at Step 3.

lunge
warrior

Lunge Warrior provides a powerful stretch through the thigh and hip of the back leg, extends the spine, and opens the chest. Feel the energy building as you breathe deeply into the ribcage.

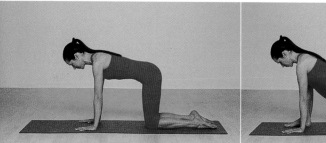

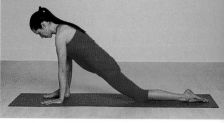

1 Begin on all fours with the hands directly beneath the shoulders and the knees beneath the hips. With fingers spread, press the palms to the floor, stretch through the arms, and bring the shoulders away from the ears.

2 As you exhale, take your right leg forward between your hands, so your knee is directly above the heel of your right foot. If necessary, come up onto your fingertips.

TAKE CARE
• If you have back problems, stop at Step 3 or 4 to begin with.
• Do not take the neck back at Step 6 if you have neck problems.
• If you have heart problems or HBP, stop at Step 4 or 5 and hold the position briefly.

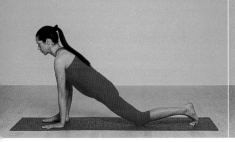

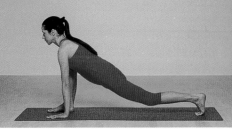

3 Tuck the toes of the left foot under and step the foot back a little. Let the right buttock sink toward the floor. Raise your head to look at the floor in front of you.

4 As you breathe in, extend the left heel backward and, for a stronger stretch, bring the knee off the floor. Lengthen through the upper body and look straight ahead.

5 Letting the knee hover just above the ground, place your hands on your right thigh and, as you breathe in, peel your upper body up, hingeing at the hip. Breathe steadily.

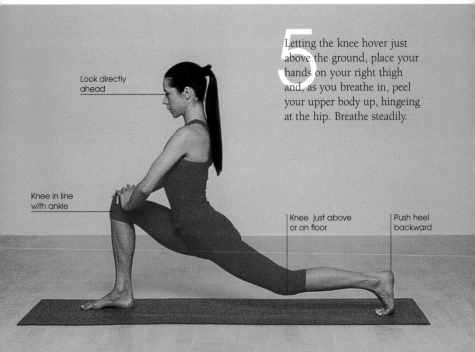

Look directly ahead

Knee in line with ankle

Knee just above or on floor

Push heel backward

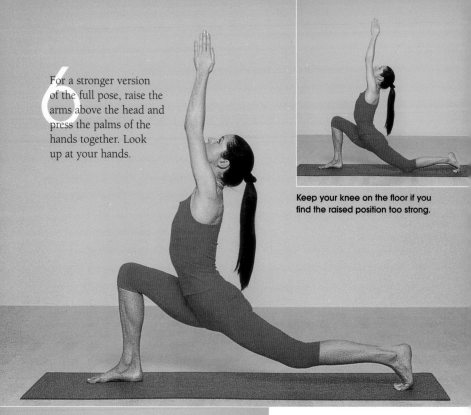

6 For a stronger version of the full pose, raise the arms above the head and press the palms of the hands together. Look up at your hands.

Keep your knee on the floor if you find the raised position too strong.

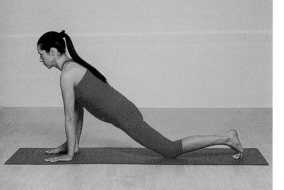

7 On an out-breath, fold forward and lower your hands to the floor on each side of your right foot. Bring your left knee to the floor. Gaze at the floor slightly ahead.

Come onto the front of your left foot. Look down at the floor and move your hips back to stretch through the back of the right leg. You may need to let your hands slide back as you move the hips back.

On an out-breath, take your right foot back to come into an all-fours position again. Your wrists should be positioned directly below your shoulders and your knees aligned with your hips. Look down at the floor.

Keeping your hands still, sit back on your heels on an out-breath, feeling the stretch through the spine. Relax the arms and stay for several breaths. Repeat Steps 1 to 9 on the left side of the body.

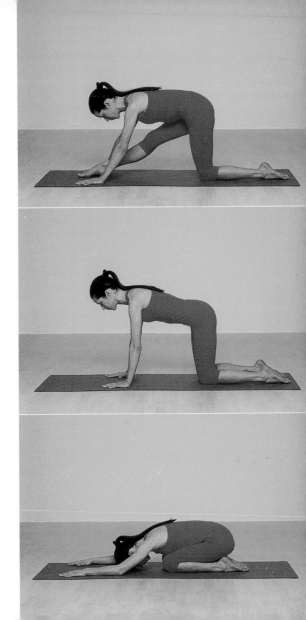

downward
dog

This calming inversion balances the upper and lower body. Keep your weight moving up and back, your shoulders broad and soft, as you stretch from the base of your fingers to your sitting bones.

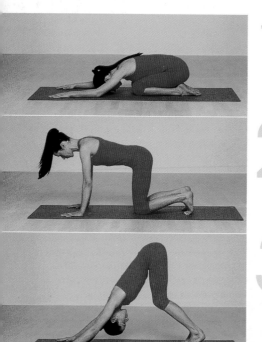

1 Sit on your heels with your legs hip-width apart. Fold your body forward on an out-breath. Stretch your arms forward and spread the fingers.

2 Breathing in, come up onto all fours, with the knees beneath the hips, the feet hip-width apart, and the hands shoulder-width apart. Press the palms into the floor and stretch through the arms. Tuck your toes under.

3 On an out-breath, lift your hips up and back. Keeping your knees bent, take your weight back toward your feet to lengthen through the spine. If your shoulders are tight, take your hands farther forward or your feet back to lengthen through the spine.

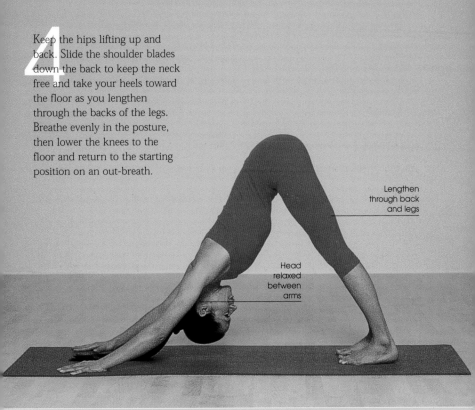

4 Keep the hips lifting up and back. Slide the shoulder blades down the back to keep the neck free and take your heels toward the floor as you lengthen through the backs of the legs. Breathe evenly in the posture, then lower the knees to the floor and return to the starting position on an out-breath.

Lengthen
through back
and legs

Head
relaxed
between
arms

ALTERNATIVES

If you have HBP, a heart condition, glaucoma, or a detached retina, do the posture with your hands resting on a chair seat or back. If you have a back problem, do the posture cautiously with your knees bent throughout.

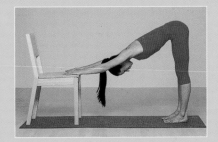

crocodile

This challenging static posture uses muscles in the arms, back, abdomen, and legs to keep the body balanced and still. In the posture, stay focused and visualize the body floating above the floor.

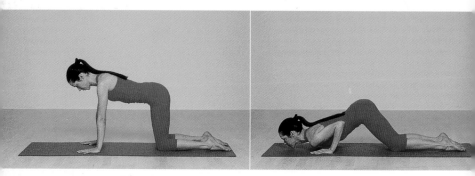

1 Start on all fours with your knees beneath your hips, your hands a little in front of your shoulders, and your feet hip-width apart. Look down. Take several breaths.

2 On an out-breath, bend your arms and lower your upper body toward the floor. Stop when your chest is a few inches above the floor. Keep your elbows tucked in close to the side of your body.

TAKE CARE
If you are very overweight, or have HBP or a heart condition, hold the full pose for a short time only or try the alternative posture (right).

3 Breathing in, tuck your toes under and lift your knees off the floor. Take the top of your chest forward, so that your elbows are above your wrists. Pull your abdomen back toward the spine, so your whole body is parallel to the floor. Step your feet back if you need to.

Upper arms parallel to floor

Extend heels back

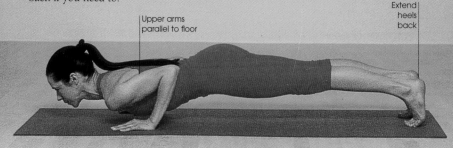

4 To come out of the pose, lower the knees back to the floor on an out-breath. Then slowly lower the rest of the body to the floor. Rest with your head on the backs of your hands. Come back into the all-fours position and repeat the sequence once.

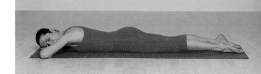

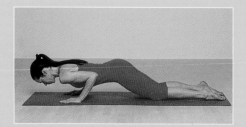

ALTERNATIVE

If you cannot hold your body parallel to the floor in the final position, practice with your knees on the floor until you are stronger.

upward
dog

This posture gives a powerful upward lift through the front of the body, extending the spine and opening the chest to encourage ribcage breathing. It gives you a feeling of strength and vitality.

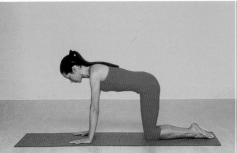 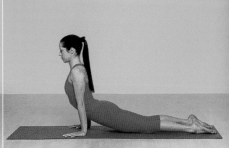

1 Start on your hands and knees, arms shoulder-width apart, feet and knees a little apart. Spread your fingers, with the middle finger pointing directly ahead. Take several breaths.

2 Breathe in deeply and, as you breathe out, allow your hips to sink forward and down. Keep your arms straight, insides of elbows facing each other, and look straight ahead. Roll the shoulders back and down.

TAKE CARE
- If you have HBP or a heart condition, hold the posture for short time only.
- Stretch forward cautiously if you have a hernia, or have had recent abdominal surgery, or suffer back pain.

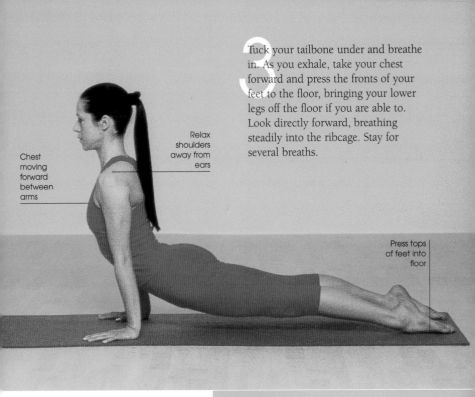

Chest moving forward between arms

Relax shoulders away from ears

3 Tuck your tailbone under and breathe in. As you exhale, take your chest forward and press the fronts of your feet to the floor, bringing your lower legs off the floor if you are able to. Look directly forward, breathing steadily into the ribcage. Stay for several breaths.

Press tops of feet into floor

4 To come out of the pose, bend the arms to lower yourself to the floor. Lie on your front, arms beside your body, palms facing up, resting with your head turned to the side.

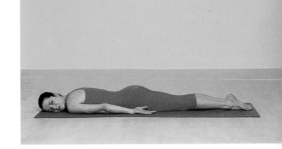

sun salute

This dynamic sequence energizes the whole body system. Focus on coordinating movement with breath and making the sequence fluid. Repeat three times at first, building up in multiples of three.

1 Stand up straight with your feet together, and your palms together in prayer position in front of your chest. Look straight ahead. Center yourself and then inhale fully.

2 As you exhale, open the palms and lower your hands to bring the arms to the sides of the body. Gently stretch the fingers toward the floor.

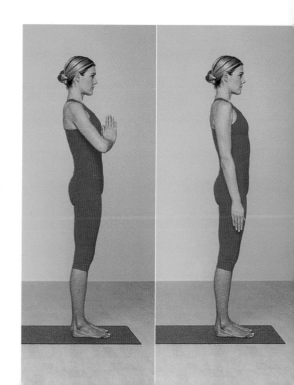

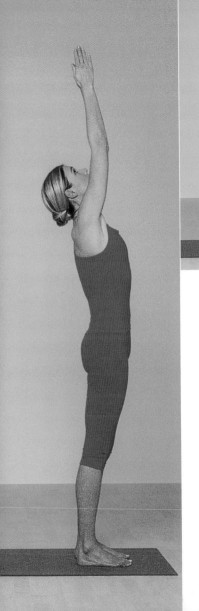

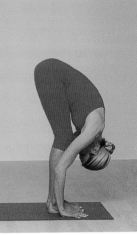

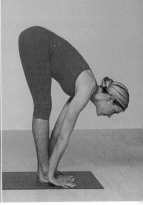

As you inhale, turn the palms out and circle your arms out to the side and up above your head. Bring your palms together and stretch up as you slightly arch backward. Look up at your hands.

Exhale, bending at the knees and hingeing forward from the hips into a relaxed Forward Bend (see p.38). Place your hands (or fingertips, if less flexible) on the floor.

Inhale as you lengthen through the backs of the legs and through the spine, drawing your upper body away from your thighs. Look at the floor slightly ahead of you. ▶

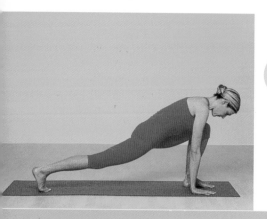

6 Exhale, bending at the knees, and take a large step back with your right foot. Land on the ball of the right foot. Your upper torso is resting on your left thigh. Look down at the floor.

7 Inhale, coming into the basic Lunge Warrior position (see p.42). Extend through the front of the body and look straight ahead.

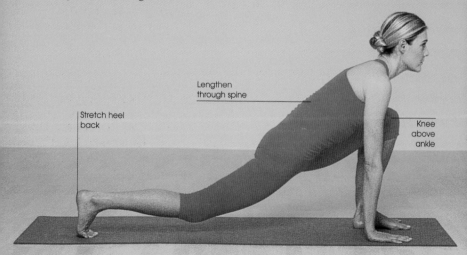

Lengthen through spine

Stretch heel back

Knee above ankle

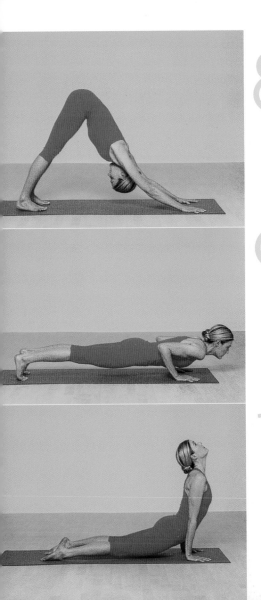

8 Exhale as you step the left foot back to come into Downward Dog (see p.46). Press your heels toward the floor, but do not force them to the floor. If necessary, keep your knees bent.

9 Holding the breath out, lower yourself into Crocodile (see p.48). Keep your heels pushing back and your abdomen drawn back toward your spine. (For an alternative way of moving from Step 8 to Step 10, see page 57.)

10 Inhale as you come into Upward Dog (see p.50). Roll over onto the fronts of your feet, extending through the front of the body and lifting the breastbone. Look up toward the ceiling. ▶

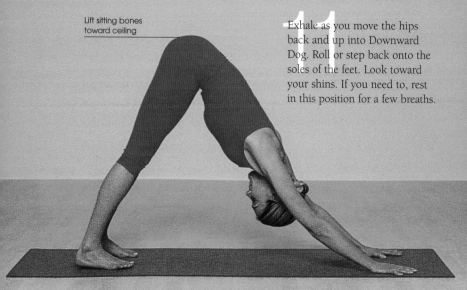

Lift sitting bones toward ceiling

11 Exhale as you move the hips back and up into Downward Dog. Roll or step back onto the soles of the feet. Look toward your shins. If you need to, rest in this position for a few breaths.

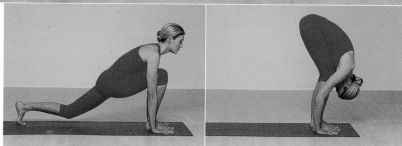

12 Inhale as you step the right foot forward between your hands to move back into Lunge Warrior, coming up onto your fingertips if you need to. If you are very stiff, you may need to take two steps forward.

13 As you exhale, bring your left foot forward to join the right foot and come into an easy Forward Bend, with bent legs if necessary. Relax your shoulders and neck.

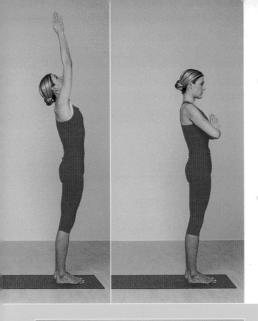

14 Inhale to come up, keeping your knees bent. As you lift up, circle your arms out to the side and bring the palms together above your head, arching the back slightly. Look up at your hands.

15 Exhale as you lower your arms to bring the palms in front of the chest in prayer position. Lower the head to look directly ahead. Repeat the sequence, taking the left leg back at Step 6. This constitutes one round.

ALTERNATIVE SUB-SEQUENCE

If you find the movements from Step 8 to 10 too strong, try the following more gentle version.

• From Downward Dog, hold the breath out and bring your knees to the floor to come onto all fours.

• Without breathing in, lower yourself to the floor with the hands underneath the shoulders, and the elbows tucked in.

• As you inhale, lift the head and shoulders and extend the top of the chest forward to come into modified Upward Dog with the fronts of the legs on the floor.

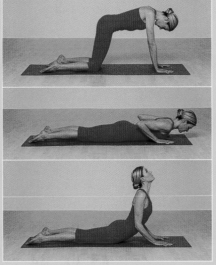

triangle

This side-bending posture helps to increase hip-joint flexibility and opens the chest. Feel the energy radiating out from the core of your body. Do not worry if your lower hand is a long way from the floor.

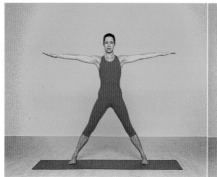
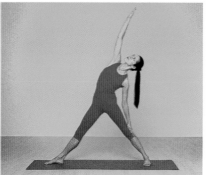

1 Stand with your feet 3 ft (1 m) or more apart, palms together in front of your chest. Look forward. As you breathe in, sweep your arms up and out to the side at shoulder level.

2 Turn your left heel out a little and rotate the right leg out until your toes point to the side. Drop the left arm onto the leg and stretch the right arm up. Take several breaths.

TAKE CARE
• If you have back problems, rest front arm higher up the leg.
• Do not turn your head to look up at your hand if you have neck problems.

As you breathe out, reach out sideways over the right leg. At the same time, slide your left hand up to bring the palm against the small of your back. Look along your right arm. Feel your spine lengthen, your chest and hips open to the front.

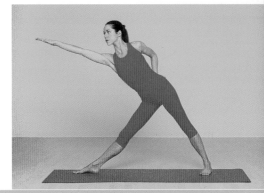

Bring the right hand to the floor or to wherever is comfortable on your leg, and turn your head to look forward. Take your left arm up toward the ceiling, palm facing forward. Keeping the back of your neck aligned with your spine, look up at your left hand. Come up on an in-breath and repeat on the left side.

Keep upper body lifted, chest open

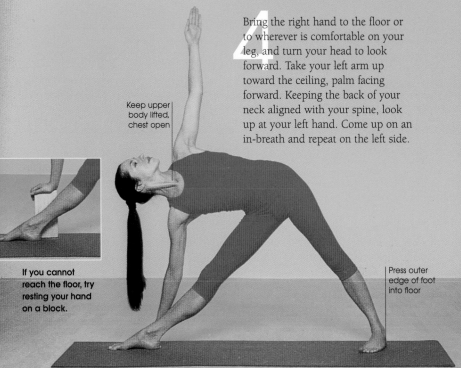

If you cannot reach the floor, try resting your hand on a block.

Press outer edge of foot into floor

bent-knee
side bend

This sideways-bending posture gives an invigorating stretch through the upper side of the body, while opening the hips and the chest. Keep the back leg strong, and the front hip, knee, and foot in line.

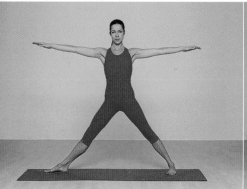 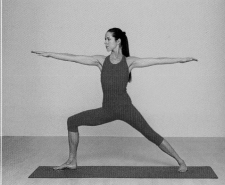

1 Stand with your feet about 3 ft (1 m) or more apart, palms together in front of your chest. As you breathe in, sweep your arms up and out to the sides at shoulder level, palms facing the floor. Turn your left heel out slightly, and rotate the right leg and foot 90 degrees to the right.

2 Breathe in deeply; then, as you exhale, bend the right knee to the side until the knee is above the heel. Turn the upper torso to look along the right arm and feel your tailbone dropping toward the floor. Hold, taking a couple of breaths.

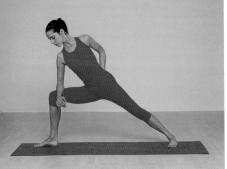

On an exhalation, bend to the right, bringing the right forearm to rest on the right thigh. Bring the palm of the left hand on to your sacrum. Open the chest to the front and press the outside edges of the feet to the floor. Look down at your right knee.

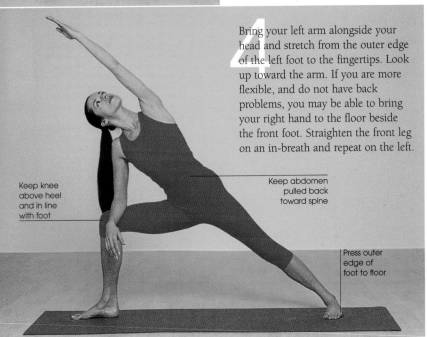

Bring your left arm alongside your head and stretch from the outer edge of the left foot to the fingertips. Look up toward the arm. If you are more flexible, and do not have back problems, you may be able to bring your right hand to the floor beside the front foot. Straighten the front leg on an in-breath and repeat on the left.

Keep knee above heel and in line with foot

Keep abdomen pulled back toward spine

Press outer edge of foot to floor

TAKE CARE
• Look straight ahead if you have neck problems. • Keep your forearm on the thigh and your hand on your back if you have HBP.

runners'
stretch

Called Runners' Stretch because it works particularly on the hamstrings and calf muscles of the leading leg, this posture also massages and helps tone your digestive organs with every breath.

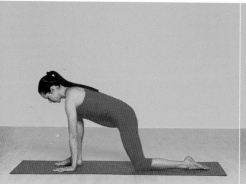 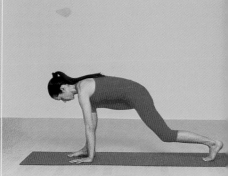

Start in the all-fours position, hands shoulder-width apart, fingers spread and pointing forward. Step your right leg forward, bringing the sole of the foot to rest between your hands, so that the knee is directly above the heel. Look down at the floor.

Lengthen your upper body forward over the right thigh. Come onto the ball of your left foot and, as you breathe in, lift your left knee away from the floor. Keep the palms of your hands flat on the floor.

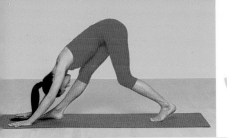

3 As you breathe out, lift the sitting bones up and back, and lengthen through the back of the right leg, keeping the left knee bent.

4 Lengthen through the upper body, keeping the back relaxed, and straightening the right leg. Straighten the left leg if the right leg is straight. Repeat on the left side.

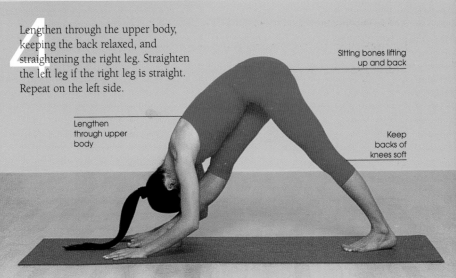

Sitting bones lifting up and back

Lengthen through upper body

Keep backs of knees soft

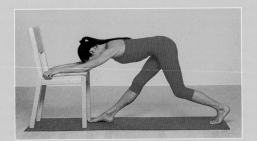

ALTERNATIVE

If you find the stretch too intense, or if you have back problems, HBP, a heart condition, glaucoma, or a detached retina, do the posture using a chair. Hold onto the seat of a chair as you bend forward. If necessary, keep the left leg bent to protect the back.

lunge
twist

This posture combines a twist for the spine with a wide arm stretch to help relieve backaches and stiffness in the shoulders. Focus on breathing smoothly and on broadening across the top of the chest.

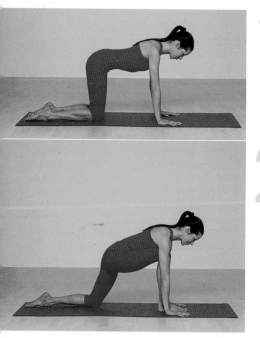

1 Start on your hands and knees, your arms shoulder-width apart. Spread your fingers, with the middle finger pointing directly ahead. Look down at the floor.

2 Bring the right foot forward and place between the hands, so the knee is directly above the ankle and the heels of the hands align with the ankle. Lengthen through the upper body.

TAKE CARE
• Twist cautiously if you have back problems or a hernia.
• If you have neck problems, do not look up.
• Rest the upper hand on the thigh of the bent leg if you have HBP.

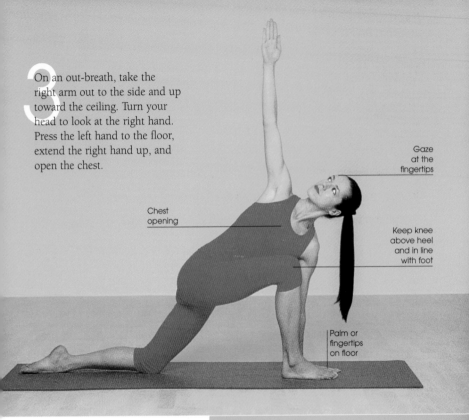

On an out-breath, take the right arm out to the side and up toward the ceiling. Turn your head to look at the right hand. Press the left hand to the floor, extend the right hand up, and open the chest.

Gaze at the fingertips

Chest opening

Keep knee above heel and in line with foot

Palm or fingertips on floor

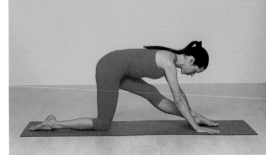

To come out from the pose, lower your right hand to the floor again and stretch through the back of the right leg. Then come back to the all-fours position. Repeat the sequence on the left side.

wide leg
forward bend

This posture provides an invigorating stretch to the backs of the legs and inner thighs. It also reverses the effect of gravity on the upper body, easing out the back and calming the mind.

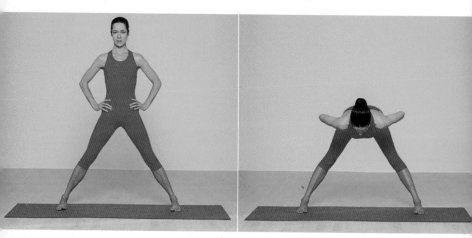

1 Stand with your legs 3 ft (1 m) or so apart, hands on hips, and feet facing forward. Look straight ahead. Draw the muscles in the fronts of the thighs up and out. Lift the breastbone. Breathe in.

2 As you breathe out, hinge forward and down from the hips, keeping the spine long. If you have a back problem, bend your knees before bending forward. Look down.

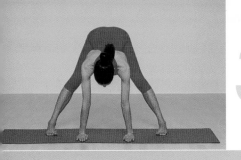

Still breathing out, bring your hands to the floor directly below the shoulders. Breathe in, pressing your hands into the floor to lengthen through the arms and back.

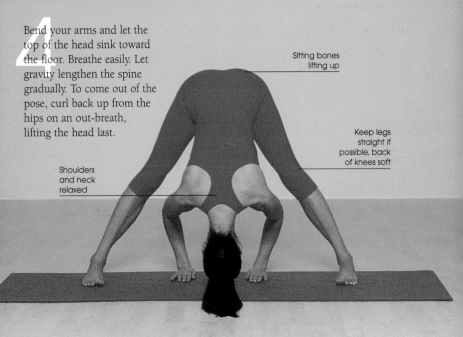

Bend your arms and let the top of the head sink toward the floor. Breathe easily. Let gravity lengthen the spine gradually. To come out of the pose, curl back up from the hips on an out-breath, lifting the head last.

Sitting bones lifting up

Keep legs straight if possible, back of knees soft

Shoulders and neck relaxed

TAKE CARE
• If you have back problems, keep the knees bent and/or use a chair for support. • Bend forward halfway, using a chair, if you have HBP, a heart condition, glaucoma, or a detached retina.

side-bending
sequence

This dynamic side-bending sequence can help you feel calm, centered, and invigorated. Try taking three breaths in each stage of the sequence to help the body open and the mind let go.

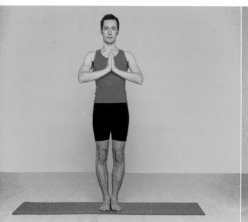

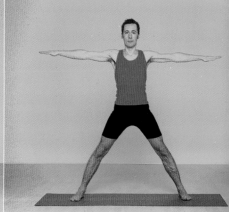

1 Stand with your feet together, hands in prayer position in front of your chest. Standing up tall, take a little time to center yourself, breathing easily and gently pressing the heels of the hands together.

2 Step your feet 3 ft (1 m) or more apart. Then sweep your arms up and out to shoulder level, palms facing down. The arms should feel active, the shoulders relaxed.

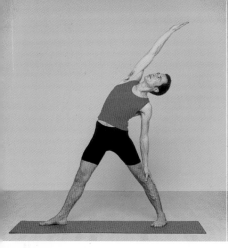

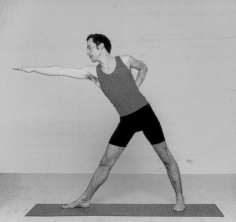

3 Turn the left heel out and rotate the right leg so the toes face the end of the mat. As you breathe in, raise the right arm and arch to the left, opening the right side of the body. Lower the left arm to rest on the left leg.

4 As you breathe out, reach out to the side with the right arm, and bring the left hand onto the lower back. Lengthen through the trunk. Look along the right arm.

5 Bring the right hand onto the right leg, as close to the ankle as you find comfortable. Press the left hand gently against the back to help open the chest. Keep the hips as open as possible. Extend through the spine, with the top of the head moving to the side wall. Look forward. ▶

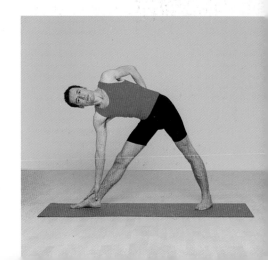

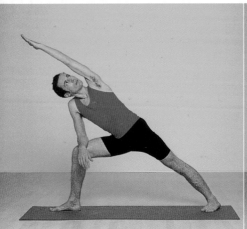

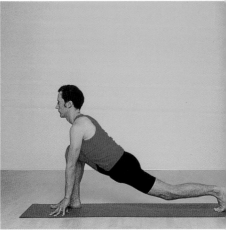

Breathing out, bend the right knee over the heel. Bring the right forearm onto the right thigh and rest it there. Stretch the left arm alongside the head. Keep the hips open and turn the head to look up at the arm.

On the out-breath, lower your left arm and bring your hands to the floor on each side of, and parallel to, the right foot. Simultaneously, pivot on the ball of your left foot to come into Lunge Warrior (see p.42).

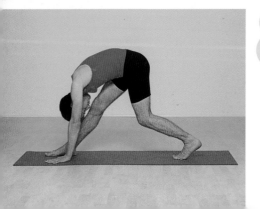

Take a step forward with the left foot to come into Runners' Stretch (see p.62). Keeping the left knee bent, stretch through the back of the right leg as much as you find comfortable. Lengthen through your upper body as you fold forward. Visualize your sitting bones moving up and back toward the top of the wall behind you. Keep your back relaxed and your hands on the floor.

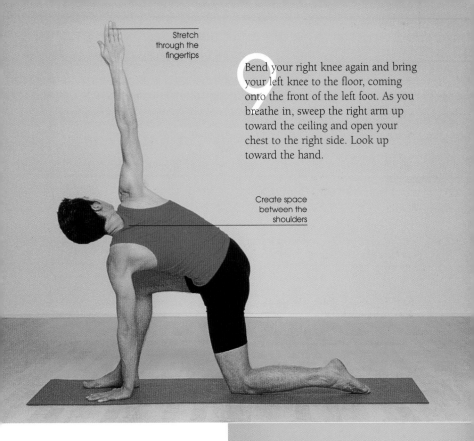

Stretch
through the
fingertips

9 Bend your right knee again and bring
your left knee to the floor, coming
onto the front of the left foot. As you
breathe in, sweep the right arm up
toward the ceiling and open your
chest to the right side. Look up
toward the hand.

Create space
between the
shoulders

10 Bring the right hand back to
the floor on an out-breath. Come
onto the ball of the left foot and
move back into Runners' Stretch.
Remember to lift the sitting bones
up and back while keeping the
upper body soft. ▶

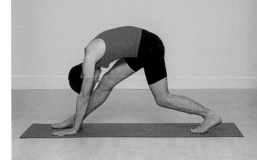

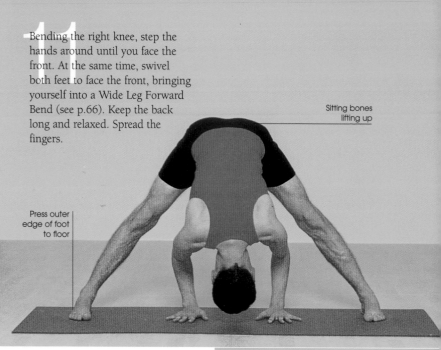

Bending the right knee, step the hands around until you face the front. At the same time, swivel both feet to face the front, bringing yourself into a Wide Leg Forward Bend (see p.66). Keep the back long and relaxed. Spread the fingers.

Sitting bones lifting up

Press outer edge of foot to floor

Bend your knees and bring your hands onto your hips. As you breathe in, keeping the back relaxed, slowly uncurl your body to come up. Stack the vertebrae up one at a time, finally raising the head to face the front and straightening the legs.

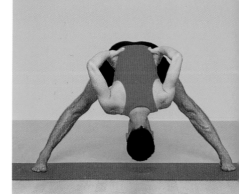

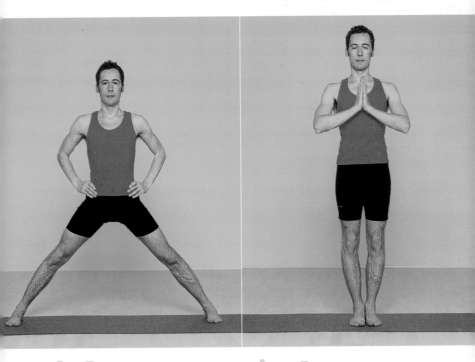

Pressing into the outside edges of the feet, rotate the thigh bones out. Press the elbows a little toward the back wall. Open and lift the chest, broadening across the front of the shoulders. Look straight ahead. Take a couple of breaths.

Step the feet together, bringing the palms together in front of the chest. Repeat the whole sequence, working on the left side of the body. Then stand quietly with your eyes closed for a short while and experience the energy and the stillness.

child

Child is a restorative pose that gently stretches the spine and postural muscles in the back, while taking your attention inward. It is a good posture for developing breath awareness.

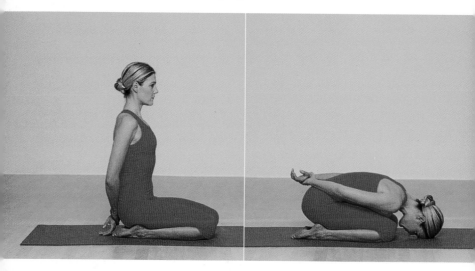

1 Kneel and sit back on your heels, looking straight ahead. With your hands behind your back, hold one wrist with the other hand. Lengthen through the spine. Breathe in.

2 As you exhale, fold forward over the knees, hingeing from the hips. Bring your forehead to the floor. (Rest your forehead on a block or other support if this is difficult.)

3 Bring your arms to the floor alongside the body, or, as shown, beside the head. Rest in the pose, focusing on breathing quietly and steadily. Child can also be done dynamically (if you do not suffer from epilepsy), moving alternately between Step 1 and 2 with the breath five to 10 times.

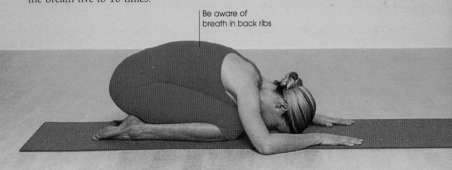

Be aware of
breath in back ribs

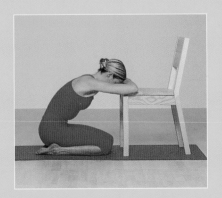

ALTERNATIVE

If you have back problems, HBP, glaucoma, or a detached retina, do not bring the head to the floor. Instead, rest your head on your hands with your forearms on the seat of a chair.

hare

Like Child, Hare is a restorative pose; it stretches the spine and helps relieve stiffness in the shoulder girdle. Try to let the spine lengthen and the shoulders relax on the out-breath.

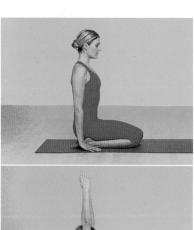

1 Sit up straight, sitting back on your heels. Press your hands into the mat on each side of your torso, fingers pointing forward. Lengthen through the spine and look straight ahead.

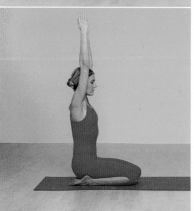

2 On an in-breath, circle your arms out to the sides of your body and up above your head. Lower them on the out-breath, and raise them again on the in-breath.

TAKE CARE
If you have back problems, glaucoma, or a detached retina, stretch forward with your hands on a chair.

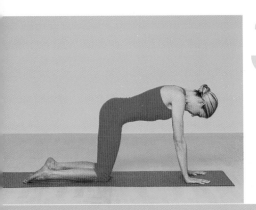

As you exhale, lower your arms forward to come onto your hands and knees. Your hands should be shoulder-width apart and your knees under your hips.

On an exhalation, keeping your hands still, take your hips back to sit on your heels. Feel the stretch through the shoulders and the back, creeping the hands forward to increase the stretch. Take several deep, slow breaths. Relax the arms and sit back up on an in-breath.

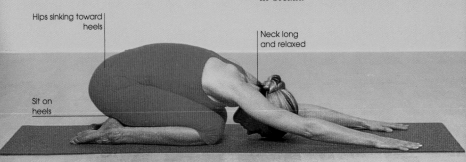

Hips sinking toward heels

Neck long and relaxed

Sit on heels

camel

Feel the energy surge through your upper body in this invigorating, back-bending posture. Lift up through the front of the body and let the tailbone drop as you arch back, to create space in the spine.

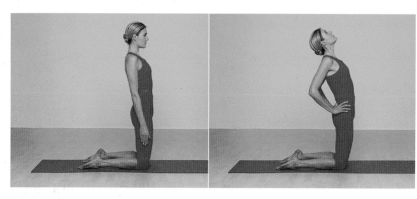

1 Kneel with the body upright and the legs hip-width apart. Press the hands against the thighs, tuck the tailbone under, and draw the abdomen in. Lift the breastbone; relax the shoulders.

2 Place your hands on your hips. As you breathe in, lift the chest, take the elbows back, and look up toward the ceiling. Exhale and hold the position as you continue to breathe steadily.

TAKE CARE
• Be very cautious going beyond Step 2 if you have back problems, a hernia, recent abdominal surgery, HBP, or heart disease.
• If you have neck problems, do not take your head back at Step 4.

3 As you breathe in, circle your right arm forward and up beside your head, and as you exhale, circle it back down to your right heel. Repeat with the left arm.

4 Keeping the thighs perpendicular, lengthen the front of the body as you slowly arch back to touch your heels. Hold for three to five breaths. Breathe in, release the hands, and come back up to kneeling upright.

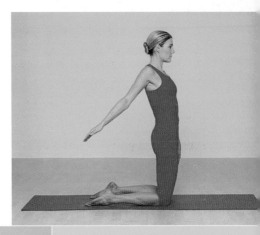

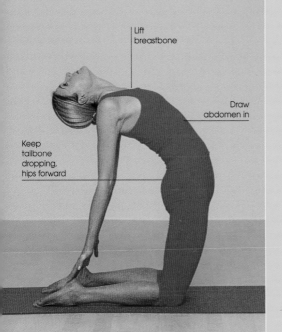

Lift breastbone

Draw abdomen in

Keep tailbone dropping, hips forward

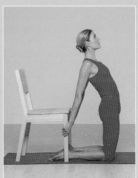

ALTERNATIVE

If your body is stiff, do not try to bring your arms right down to your heels. Instead, position a chair over your feet and lean back to hold onto its legs as far down as is comfortable.

shoulder stand
against a wall

A rejuvenating posture that reverses the effects of gravity on the body and stimulates the brain's balance centers. You may need to use a blanket under the shoulders (see p.84) to keep the neck free.

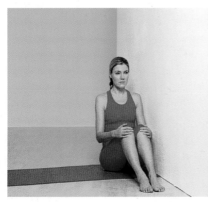

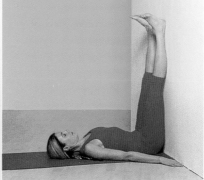

1 Sit up straight alongside a wall with your knees bent and your left hip against the wall. Take several breaths to center yourself.

2 Swivel around, supporting yourself with your hands, to lie on your back with your buttocks against the wall and your legs up the wall. Draw your shoulders away from your ears.

TAKE CARE
• Stop at Step 2 if you are seriously overweight or menstruating, or have neck problems, HBP, a heart condition, or a detached retina.
• If you have back problems, lie with your knees bent over a chair.

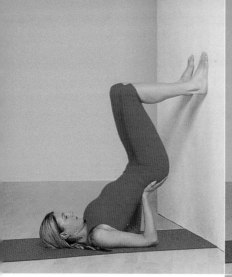

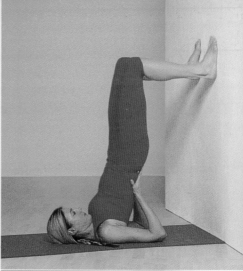

3 Bend your knees to bring the soles of the feet against the wall. Breathe in and push against the wall to lift your bottom off the floor. Support your back with your hands.

4 Keep pushing against the wall to lengthen through the front of the body until your back and thighs are perpendicular. If you feel any discomfort in the neck, come down and seek advice before trying again.

5 Make sure you are breathing easily. Lift the left leg away from the wall and point the foot straight up to the ceiling. Bring it back to the wall and do the same with the right leg. ▶

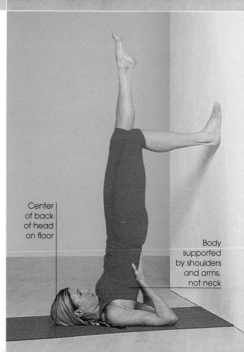

Center of back of head on floor

Body supported by shoulders and arms, not neck

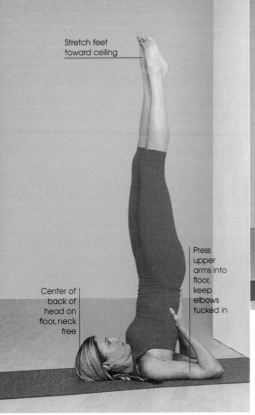

Stretch feet
toward ceiling

Center of
back of
head on
floor, neck
free

Press
upper
arms into
floor,
keep
elbows
tucked in

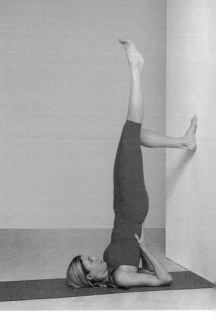

7

To come out of the pose, bend
your left knee to bring the sole
of your left foot back to the wall.
Keep stretching up through the
spine. Continue to support your
back with your hands.

6

Bring one leg and then the other
away from the wall to come into a full
Shoulder Stand. Slide your hands closer
to your shoulders to help keep the body
upright. Hold for about 30 seconds to
start with, increasing the time as you
become more familiar with the pose.
Breathe normally, stretching the feet
toward the ceiling and lengthening
through the body.

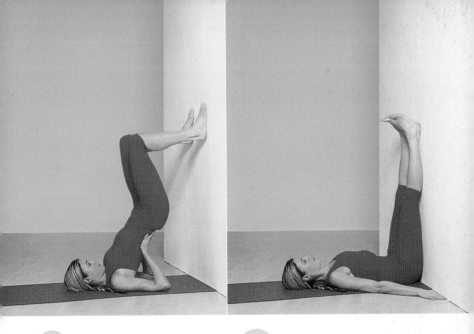

Bend your right knee to bring your right foot to the wall. Breathing normally, start to lower your spine to the floor, keeping the back supported as you come down.

When your lower back is on the floor, take your arms out to the side and stay in the position for a few breaths with your legs stretched up the wall.

On an out-breath, roll over onto your right side with your knees bent. Stay there for a short while, breathing easily. Try Easy Fish (see p.88) before moving on to practice any other postures.

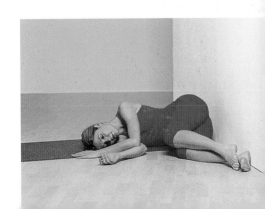

full shoulder stand

If you find Shoulder Stand Against a Wall easy, try the full version. In the final position, focus on lifting up through the spine and stretching the legs up. Keep relaxed and breathe smoothly and deeply.

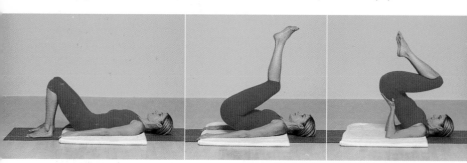

1 Lie on a folded blanket with your knees bent and your arms by your side, palms facing down. The back of the head and neck should be off the blanket.

2 On an inhalation, bend your knees over your chest and swing the legs up. Press strongly into the floor with your hands and forearms.

3 Bring your hands up to support your back, keeping your upper arms on the floor. Press your hands into the back to bring your weight onto the tops of your shoulders, making sure your neck is free and relaxed.

TAKE CARE
• As for Shoulder Stand Against a Wall. • When using a blanket, make sure the tops of the shoulders line up with the edge of the blanket and the neck is off the blanket and free.

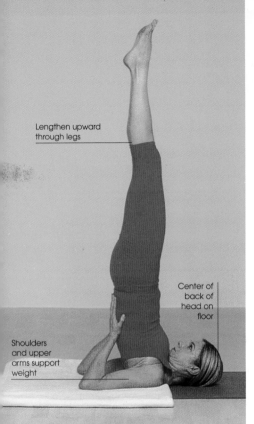

Lengthen upward through legs

Center of back of head on floor

Shoulders and upper arms support weight

4 Pushing your upper arms and elbows into the floor, slide your hands toward your shoulders to bring your upper body vertical. Slowly straighten your legs toward the ceiling and bring the elbows closer together. Breathe easily. Stay only for a short time to begin with.

5 On an exhalation, bend the knees toward the head and roll down, supporting the back with the hands. You may need to let your head and shoulders come off the floor as you roll down.

6 Come into a relaxed sitting Forward Bend with knees bent, as shown here, or simply lie on your back with your knees bent for a few breaths.

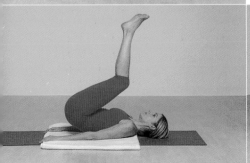

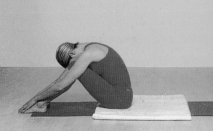

plow

A soothing pose, Plow combines some of the benefits of an inversion with a strong stretch through the upper back and the back of the legs. Avoid altogether if you have neck problems.

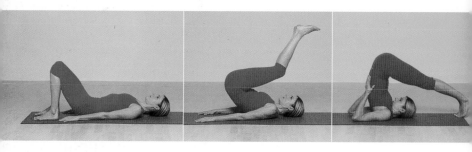

1 Lie on your back with your knees bent, feet hip-width apart. Place your arms beside your body, palms facing down. Take several breaths.

2 On an inhalation, bend the knees over the chest and swing the legs up. Press strongly into the ground with your hands and forearms.

3 Bring your hands up to support your back, keeping your upper arms on the floor as for Full Shoulder Stand (see p.84). Bring your weight onto the tops of your shoulders, making sure your neck is free and relaxed. Stretch your legs back and bring your feet to the floor.

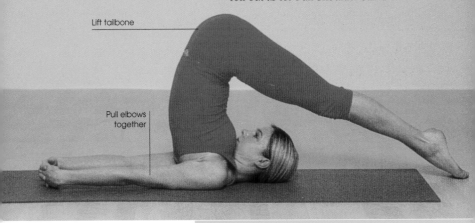

4 Lengthen up through your spine and stretch your arms out along the floor behind you with the fingers interlocked. Stay in the pose for a short while to begin with, breathing quietly. Then bend the legs again and, supporting your back, roll out as for Full Shoulder Stand.

Lift tailbone

Pull elbows together

TAKE CARE
• If you are seriously overweight, or are menstruating, have HBP, a heart condition, or a detached retina, stop at Step 3; relax and breathe easily.
• Lie on your back with knees bent over a chair if you have back problems.

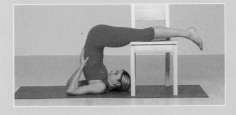

ALTERNATIVE
If you cannot reach the floor with your feet, bend your knees toward your forehead or practice with your thighs resting on a chair, as shown. Support your back with your hands.

easy fish

This posture provides an excellent counterstretch for the back and the neck after doing the Full Shoulder Stand (see p.84). Easy Fish stretches the front of the body, opens the chest, extends the spine, and strengthens the upper arms.

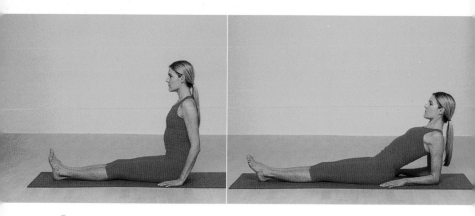

1 Sit up straight with your legs stretched out in front of you, feet together. Place your arms down by your sides. Look straight ahead. Push into the hands to lengthen through the upper body.

2 Lean back on your forearms with your elbows positioned underneath your shoulders, fingers pointing forward. Keep looking straight ahead.

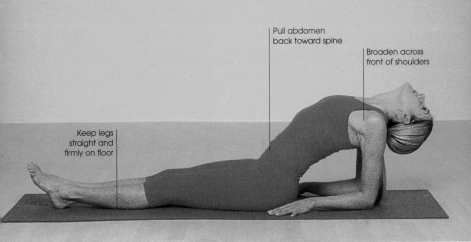

Pull abdomen
back toward spine

Broaden across
front of shoulders

Keep legs
straight and
firmly on floor

Stretch your toes away. Breathing in, press your forearms down and open your chest toward the ceiling. Slowly take your head back to look up at the ceiling, arching your back gently. Breathe deeply into the chest.

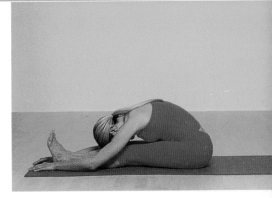

TAKE CARE
• Keep the head in line with your spine if you have neck problems.
• Do not arch the back excessively if you have back problems.

To come out of the pose, bring your head forward, then press into the forearms and hands to sit up. Fold forward, resting your forehead on your knees. If you need to, bend your knees.

sitting
forward stretch

This energy-balancing posture encourages flexibility in the spine and stretches the hamstrings, while allowing the mind to settle on your inner awareness as you relax forward.

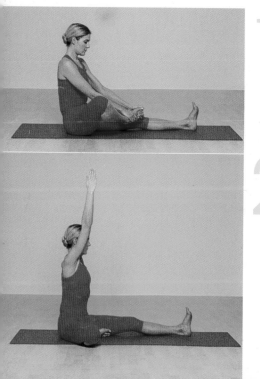

1 Sit with your feet stretched out in front of you. Press your hands into the floor at the sides of your hips to bring yourself onto your sitting bones. Then bring the sole of your right foot onto the inside of your left thigh, close to the groin.

2 Allow the right knee to sink to the floor. Bring your right hip forward to align yourself with your left leg. If your knee is a long way off the floor, support it with a pillow. As you breathe in, bring your arms up beside your head. Look straight ahead.

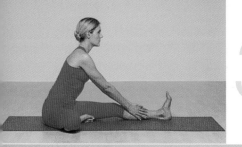

3 As you breathe out, hinge forward from the hips. Keep the back long and your gaze straight ahead. Bring your hands onto your leg. Breathe in, lengthening through the spine.

4 As you breathe out, lengthen forward again and, if you are able to, hold onto your left foot. Bend the elbows to gently bring the upper body closer to the leg without straining the back. Relax, breathing easily. Sit up slowly on an in-breath and repeat on the other side.

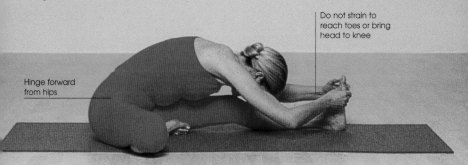

Do not strain to reach toes or bring head to knee

Hinge forward from hips

ALTERNATIVE

If you have tight hamstrings, inflexible hips or back, or a hernia, try sitting on a block, or place a folded blanket under the bent leg as you reach forward. If necessary, hold onto a belt that is looped around the foot, to avoid straining your back.

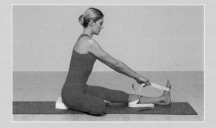

supine
butterfly

This relaxing posture can help release tension in the abdomen and pelvic area and relieve period pains. The benefits are enhanced by practicing Abdominal Breathing (see p.101) in the pose.

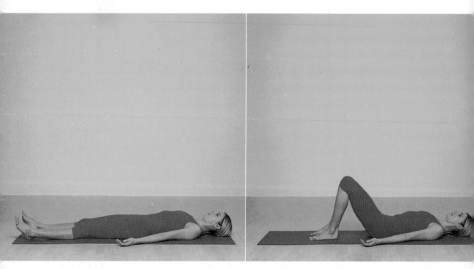

1 Lie on your back with your legs stretched out and your arms away to the sides of the body, the backs of the hands on the floor. Lengthen through the back of your neck.

2 Bend your knees, sliding your feet close to your buttocks. Feel yourself broadening across the top of the chest as you draw the shoulders down away from the ears.

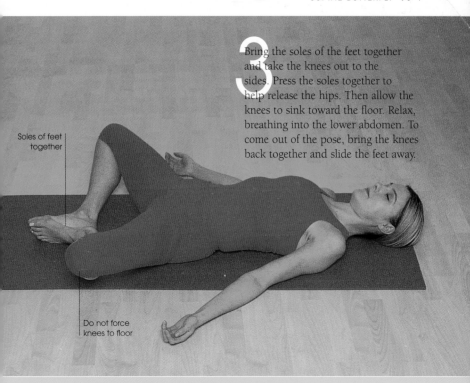

3 Bring the soles of the feet together and take the knees out to the sides. Press the soles together to help release the hips. Then allow the knees to sink toward the floor. Relax, breathing into the lower abdomen. To come out of the pose, bring the knees back together and slide the feet away.

Soles of feet together

Do not force knees to floor

ALTERNATIVE

Do not try to force the knees to the floor. If your knees do not reach the floor, or if you suffer from sacroiliac back pain, support the legs with pillows or folded blankets. To focus on Abdominal Breathing, try placing your hands on the abdomen.

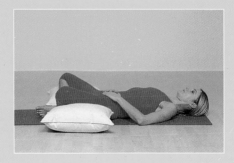

kneeling stretch
sequence

This is a calming sequence that helps you unwind and balance your energy. It is especially beneficial at the end of a stressful day, when it will refresh your mind and body, enabling you to enjoy the evening.

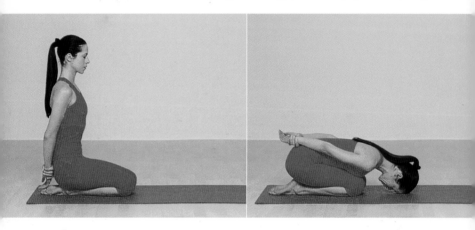

1 Sit back on your heels and hold onto your right wrist with your left hand. Lengthening through the spine and back of the neck, look straight ahead. Take several breaths with your eyes closed to center yourself. Breathe in.

2 As you breathe out, fold forward to bring the upper body onto the thighs. Breathe in and come back up to sitting. Then, as you breathe out, fold forward again.

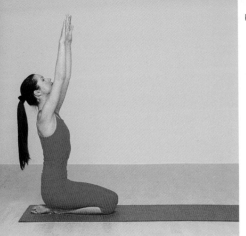

Breathing in, sit up. At the same time, circle your arms out to the side and up above your head. Look up at your fingertips.

Keeping your arms raised, fold forward on the out-breath. With your arms out in front, in line with your shoulders, gently stretch through the spine.

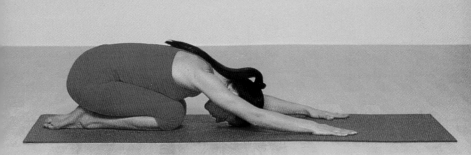

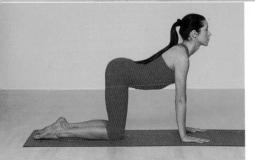

As you breathe in, come up onto all fours. Make sure your legs are hip-width apart and your wrists in line with your shoulders. Breathe out, then breathe in and tilt the tailbone up, taking the top of the chest forward as you look directly to the front. ▶

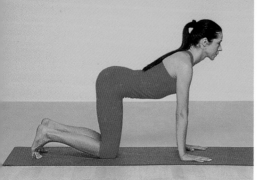

Breathe out. Then, as you breathe in, tuck your toes under. Make sure the insides of your elbows are facing each other, your hands are parallel, and your fingers point forward. Look straight ahead.

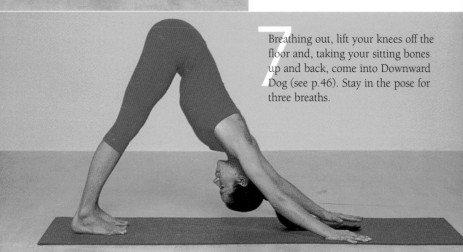

Breathing out, lift your knees off the floor and, taking your sitting bones up and back, come into Downward Dog (see p.46). Stay in the pose for three breaths.

Breathing out, come down into an all-fours position again. Lengthen through the arms and keep the shoulders down away from the ears. Look down at the floor. Breathe in and come onto the front of the feet.

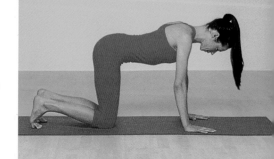

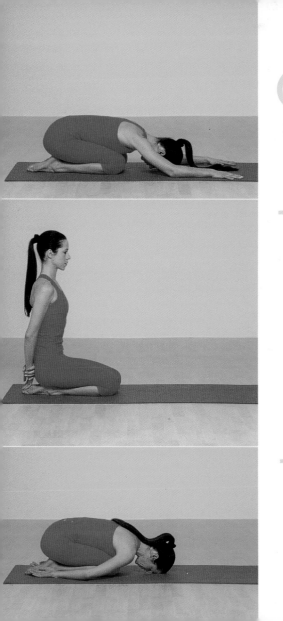

9 Keeping your hands still, take the hips back to sit on your heels as you breathe out. Stretch through the spine and relax the forearms to the floor.

10 On the in-breath, sit up, keeping the back straight. Bring your arms behind you, and hold your right wrist with your left hand. Lift though the spine and the front of the body, broadening across the top of the chest.

11 Breathing out, fold forward over the thighs to bring the forehead to the floor. Bring your arms down by your sides, palms up. Relax in this position, breathing quietly, for one or two minutes before sitting up.

sitting twist

This simple spinal twist encourages spinal flexibility, helps relieve stiffness in the shoulders and neck, and stretches respiratory muscles. Close your eyes and focus awareness on sensations within the body.

1 Sit up straight with your feet stretched out in front of you. Pressing down with your hands, make sure you are sitting toward the front edge of your sitting bones. If you have tight hamstrings, sit on a block.

2 Draw your right foot up beside your left knee and place it on the outside of the left knee. Clasp the shin with both hands and pull against it to lengthen through the spine and the front of the body.

TAKE CARE
Twist with caution if you have back problems or a hernia, or have had recent abdominal surgery.

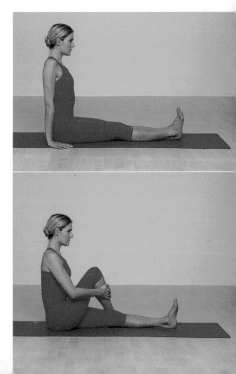

3 Take your right hand to the floor behind you and hook your left arm around your right knee. Facing forward, breathe in as you lengthen through the upper body.

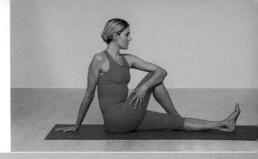

Shoulders
relaxing down

Breastbone
lifting

Hips sink
into floor

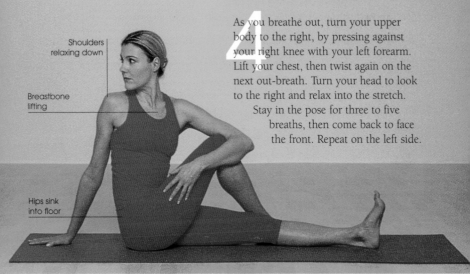

4 As you breathe out, turn your upper body to the right, by pressing against your right knee with your left forearm. Lift your chest, then twist again on the next out-breath. Turn your head to look to the right and relax into the stretch. Stay in the pose for three to five breaths, then come back to face the front. Repeat on the left side.

5 If you are more flexible, you may find it more effective to bring the back of the left arm onto the outside of the right knee. As you breathe out, keep the arm straight and pressing against the leg. Stretch the fingertips toward the floor to turn to the side.

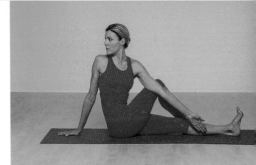

breathing
practices

The following breathing practices can be done simply to improve your awareness of the breath, but they are also particularly useful in helping to quiet the mind for meditation (see p.106).

The breathing practices described on the following six pages will help improve your breath awareness and encourage calmness and mental clarity. They are generally practiced after doing some yoga postures or some simple stretching. They help loosen up the body, so that it is easier for you to be relaxed during the breathing practices.

The practices of Mock Inhalation (see p.102) and Forced Exhalation (see p.104) are best learned with a teacher. If you have any problems, be sure to seek help.

Audible breath

A simple practice, audible breath helps make the breath smooth and even. It calms and centers the mind, and helps you to let go of tension. It can be practiced for its own sake and also during posture work, to help you remain focused.

To begin the practice, breathe through the mouth. Slightly closing the throat, make a gentle sighing "Ahhhh" sound as you breathe in and a sighing "Haaaa" sound as you breathe out.

When you have gotten a feel for this, try to achieve the same sound in the throat while breathing with your mouth closed. It may help to imagine that you are breathing through a hole in the front of the throat. Breathe smoothly and evenly, and keep your awareness on the breath. The sound of the breath can be quite subtle; only you need to hear it.

supine abdominal breathing

This practice relaxes the body and the mind, and is good for letting go of tension. Be aware of how easily the breath flows, and of the feeling of calm alertness in the mind at the end of the practice.

1 Lie on your back with your knees bent, feet about hip-width apart. Allow your breath to settle into a smooth, natural rhythm. Then become aware of the rise and fall of the abdomen as you breathe in and out. Focus on the out-breath, and very gradually allow it to become longer than the in-breath.

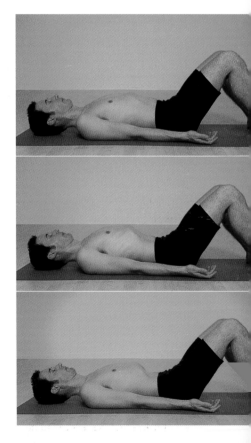

2 Make the out-breath slower and more complete by drawing the abdomen back toward the spine as you exhale. Relax as you breathe in, allowing the abdomen to swell out. Breathe like this for a while.

3 Emphasize the out-breath more by drawing up the pelvic floor muscles (as if stopping yourself from urinating). Now, as you breathe in, keep the abdomen and pelvic floor gently contracted. Feel the breath in the ribcage. As you exhale, emphasize the contraction. After a while, relax and let the breath return to normal.

mock inhalation

This practice increases awareness of the diaphragm in breathing and increases its strength and flexibility. It involves taking a full exhalation, and then closing the throat (as if you were holding your breath) and expanding the ribs as if breathing in – a "mock inhalation."

You can do mock inhalation lying on your back (see right) or standing (see below). Do three rounds of the practice, following the instructions detailed at right carefully. Breathe normally for about 20 seconds between each round. After you have completed the practice, feel the quality of the breath. If your first normal in-breath is rushed, practice mock inhalation more gently.

TAKE CARE
• Avoid if you have HBP or active inflammation or bleeding in the abdominal region.
• This practice is best avoided during menstruation, as it creates strong negative pressures in the abdomen.

ALTERNATIVE
Stand with your legs about hip-width apart, your knees slightly bent. Lean forward a little way, rounding your back slightly. Rest your hands lightly on your thighs, your elbows slightly out to the side. Follow Steps 2 and 3 shown at right.

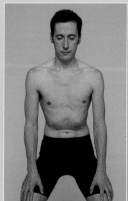
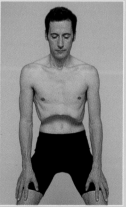

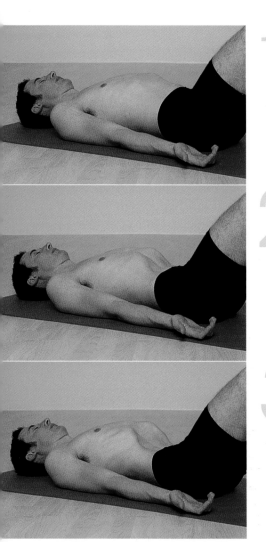

1 Lie on the floor with your knees bent, arms away from the side of the body, palms up. Allow the breath to settle into a natural, regular rhythm.

2 Breathe in deeply, allowing the abdomen to swell out. Then breathe out completely, drawing the abdomen back toward the spine at the same time.

3 Relax the abdomen, close the throat, and simultaneously expand the chest, without breathing in, to suck the abdomen up under the ribcage. Hold until you need to breathe in. To breathe in, relax the ribs first, open the throat, and contracting the abdominal muscles slightly, let the breath flow in, in a slow, controlled way.

forced exhalation

This practice involves a forced exhalation and a passive in-breath. The intense focus on the out-breath helps clear the mind of distractions and balance the nervous system.

Do three rounds, following the instructions at right carefully, and breathing naturally for about 20 seconds between each round. Maintain the same number of exhalations in each round. At the end of the third round, exhale completely and allow a short, natural pause with the breath held out. The next in-breath should be smooth and unhurried. Sit quietly, let the breath be free, and be aware of the smoothness and quietness of the breath and the mind.

During the practice, maintain a steady, even rhythm – slow down if necessary. Never try to keep going if you get out of breath. As you become more familiar with the practice, you can increase the number of exhalations per round.

BLOWING OUT THE CANDLE

This preliminary practice will help you get the feel for the correct action of the abdomen in Forced Exhalation. Rest your right hand on the abdomen and bring your left hand in front of you. Imagine that there is a candle in front of your left hand. Take half a breath in and try to blow it out. Feel the abdomen sharply contract away from your hand and then automatically relax back toward it.

Repeatedly try to blow out the candle. Then try with the mouth closed, by exhaling sharply through the nostrils.

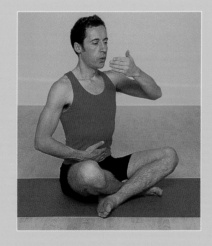

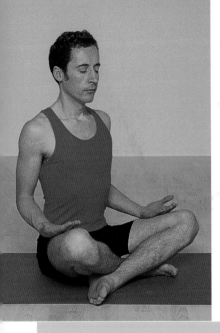

1 Sit cross-legged, spine and head erect, with your hands resting on your thighs, palms facing up. Close your eyes. Let the breath settle into a regular rhythm, emphasizing the out-breath.

2 Breathe in halfway and then exhale forcibly by sharply pulling the abdomen in. Immediately allow the abdomen to relax, so the in-breath is effortless and completely passive.

3 Repeatedly exhale, forcibly in this way up to a maximum of 10 times. This constitutes one round. Then breathe normally for 20 seconds.

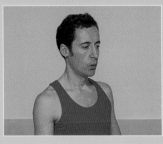

ALTERNATIVE

Sit or stand. Take a full breath in. Breathe out through the mouth in short, rapid puffs, with a brief pause between each puff, until the lungs are empty. Close your mouth and allow a natural pause with the breath held out. Then breathe in slowly and smoothly.

TAKE CARE

• If you become dizzy or breathless during the practice, stop, take a break, then try more slowly and less forcefully.
• If both nostrils are congested, you are menstruating, you have HBP, or you suffer from epilepsy, do the alternative, above.

meditation

Meditation involves silencing the mind and realizing the vital energy that constitutes the core of our being. Regular meditation has great restorative powers, helping to bring your energies into balance.

We cannot meditate by seeking to shut out the world around us or by completely ignoring our senses, thoughts, or emotions. But we can progressively let go of them, so that they do not cloud our consciousness, our awareness.

Sit comfortably in a basic sitting position (see p.19) with your head, neck, and spine erect. If you are more flexible, sit as shown opposite, with your thumb and index finger together in the mudra symbolizing the link between individual and universal energy. Be aware of your surroundings. Close your eyes and be aware of sounds and other sensations, like the touch of the air on your skin. Let the world be there without reacting to it. Become aware of your body. As you breathe out, let go of tension – in your face, your neck, your shoulders, your arms, and your legs. Be aware of your breath, which is your constant connection with the world around you. Be aware of the breath in the nostrils as you breathe in and out. Be aware of it passing through the nostrils and down

PRACTICAL MATTERS
• Choose a time when you can remain undisturbed for at least 15 minutes.
• Choose a room (or outdoor space) that is quiet, uncluttered, and not cold.
• Choose a posture – sitting or kneeling on the floor or sitting in a chair – that you will be able to sustain easily for some time.

the back of the throat to the chest as you breathe in. Feel it rising up from the chest through the back of the throat and out through the nostrils as you breathe out.

Then become aware of the space inside your head, your throat, and your neck. Be aware of the space in the right side of the chest, in the left side. Be aware of the space in the right shoulder, right arm, right hand; in the left shoulder, left arm, left hand; the space in the right hip, right leg, right foot; in the left hip, left leg, left foot. Be aware of the space above and below the navel, at the base of the spine, and in the pelvis.

Be aware of the space in the whole body. Be aware of space around the body, and the infinite space beyond. Be aware of yourself as a center of consciousness – with no separation between inside and outside. Stay with this awareness. Slowly become aware once more of your breath, your body, your surroundings.

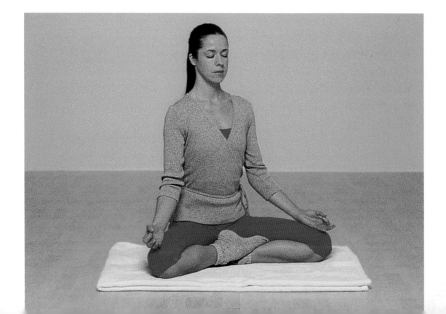

relaxation

At the end of your yoga session, stay quiet for a while to reinforce the restorative and regenerative benefits. This simple relaxation practice will take about 15 to 20 minutes. Make sure you are warm enough.

Lie on the floor, with your knees bent and your arms away from the body. Become aware of your body and how it feels. Lift your hips slightly and extend your tailbone toward your feet, and then lower the hips again, easing out the lower back. Slide your feet along the floor to stretch your legs out (unless this incurs lower back pain, in which case keep your knees bent).

Allow the legs and feet to roll outward. Tuck in your chin and then release it to bring the center of the back of your head onto the floor. If your neck feels uncomfortable like this, try resting it on a pillow or folded blanket.

Now relax your body part by part, starting with your toes and ending with your head. There is no need to do anything active, just take your attention to each part of the body in turn: feet, legs, hips, hands, arms, shoulders, torso, neck, head. Close your eyes and mouth. Be still.

Bring your attention to your breath and let it settle into a natural, regular rhythm. Do not try to breathe in any particular way; simply observe the movement of the breath in and out of the body. As you breathe in, the abdomen gently rises and as you breathe out, it sinks back down again. Gradually allow the out-breath to become a little longer than the in-breath, and be aware that as you breathe out, the body becomes a little more relaxed, a little heavier, seeming to sink into the floor.

Keeping your focus on the breath, count your breaths up to 20 and then back down again. One is an in-breath, two an out-breath, and so on. On the way down from 20, when you reach 10, only count your out-breaths until you reach zero. If you are distracted by thoughts, sounds, or other sensations, return to the breath and the counting.

When you reach zero, let go of the focus on the breath and be aware of the space in front of your eyes; the stillness and the silence. Notice how quiet the breath is, how quiet the mind is. Everything you hear and feel is taking place within your consciousness – you are aware of everything, but there is no need to focus on anything. You are wholly in the present moment – just being. Enjoy this feeling of peace and quiet for as long as it lasts.

Become aware of your body again, the floor beneath you, and the walls around you. Be aware of sounds outside and inside the room. Wriggle your toes and fingers, your hands and your feet. Take one or two deep breaths to bring more energy into the body, and then stretch your arms over your head and give a long sigh. Turn onto your right side and stay there with your eyes closed for a few moments, and then slowly sit up and open your eyes.

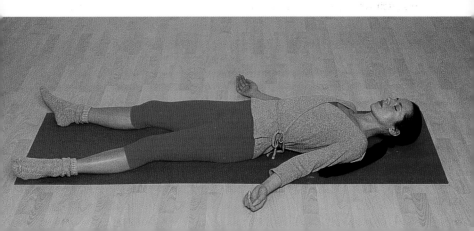

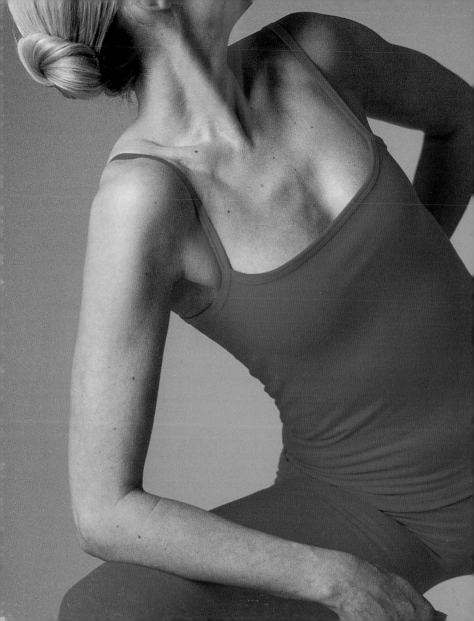

programs

Here are seven programs for those times in the day when you need a quick lift. Remember to take time to center yourself before doing them and time to absorb their effects afterward. Their benefits will be greatly enhanced if you remember that yoga is also about lifestyle and attitude.

1 start the
day right

Liven yourself up before breakfast with Sectional Breathing (see p.25) or Mock Inhalation (see p.102), some breathe-and-stretch exercises (see p.26), followed by these postures. For a more dynamic start to the day, do the Sun Salute (see p.52) before the postures. Early morning is also a good time for Meditation (see p.106).

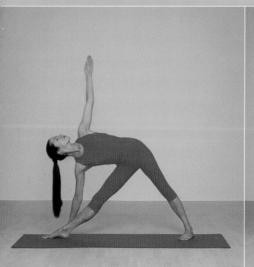

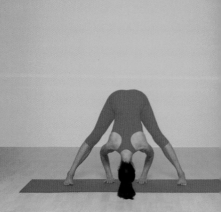

1 Triangle (see pp.58–59)

2 Wide Leg Forward Bend (pp.66–6

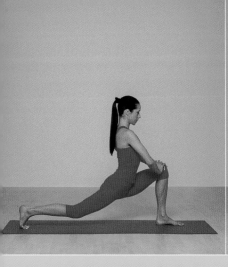

3 Lunge Warrior (see pp.42–45)

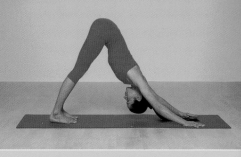

4 Downward Dog (see pp.46–47)

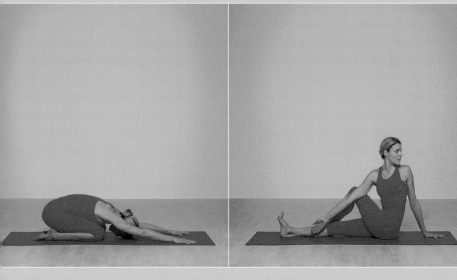

5 Hare (see pp.76–77)

6 Sitting Twist (see pp.98–99)

② midmorning
boost

Instead of grabbing a coffee, cigarette, or bagel, try these postures. In the workplace you may be able to find a quiet space to do them. If not, some breathe-and-stretch exercises (see p.26) can be done at your desk. If time is really short, Audible Breath (see p.100) or Forced Exhalation (see p.104) will leave you energized, your mind clear.

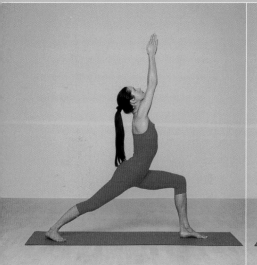

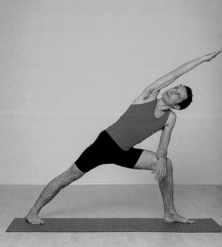

① **Warrior** (see pp.40–41)

② **Bent-Knee Side Bend** (pp.60–61)

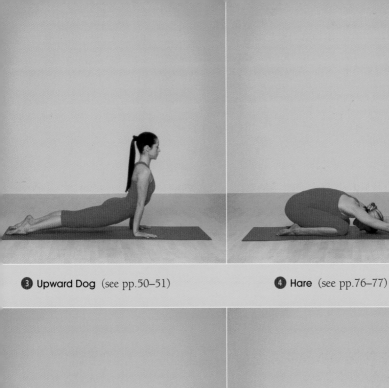

3 **Upward Dog** (see pp.50–51)

4 **Hare** (see pp.76–77)

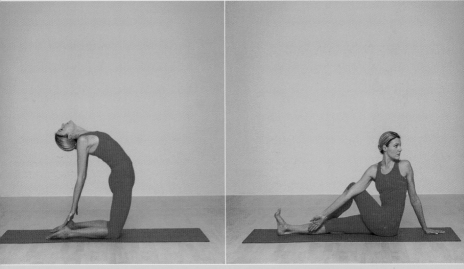

5 **Camel** (see pp.78–79)

6 **Sitting Twist** (see pp.98–99)

3 evening
recharge

After a hard day at work or a long day with the children, stretch out those tired muscles and stiff joints with these postures. Do some breathe-and-stretch exercises (see p.26) first, and practice Abdominal Breathing (see p.101) while in Supine Butterfly (see p.92), then relax. Early evening is also a good time to practice Meditation (see p.106).

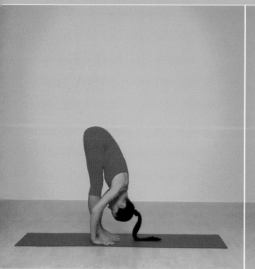

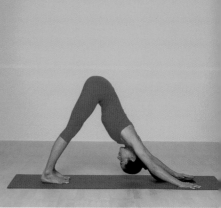

1 Forward Bend (see pp.38–39)

2 Downward Dog (see pp.46–47)

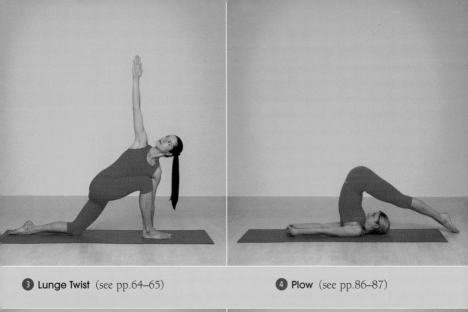

3 Lunge Twist (see pp.64–65)

4 Plow (see pp.86–87)

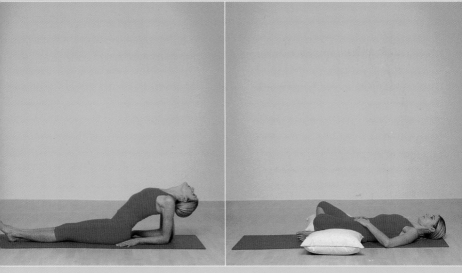

5 Easy Fish (see pp.88–89)

6 Supine Butterfly (see pp.92–93)

4 prepare for the
next day

Here is a routine to stretch the body gently and counter the pull of gravity just before going to bed. In bed, do Abdominal Breathing (see p.101) first, then relax, repeating the following affirmation: *"My energy is strong"* (with palms on abdomen, then on ribcage, then fingers on top of breastbone); *"I am ready for life"* (arms out to side).

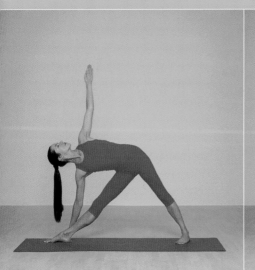

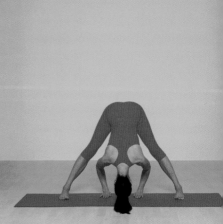

1 Triangle (see pp.58–59)

2 Wide Leg Forward Bend (pp.66–67)

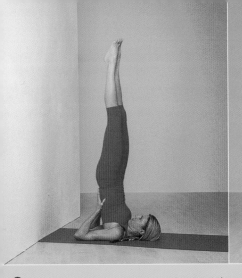

③ **Shoulder Stand Against a Wall** (pp.80–83)

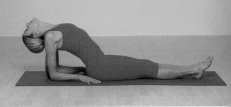

④ **Easy Fish** (see pp.88–89)

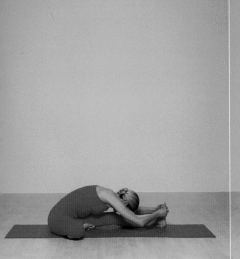

⑤ **Sitting Forward Stretch** (see pp.90–91)

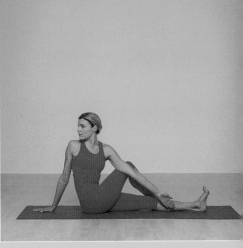

⑥ **Sitting Twist** (see pp.98–99)

⑤ midweek
boost

Here is a strong sequence to pick you up when your energy starts to flag in the middle of the week. Start with Sectional Breathing (see p.25) and some breathe-and-stretch exercises of your choice (see p.26). Then do the postures shown here. Try using Audible Breath (see p.100) throughout the program.

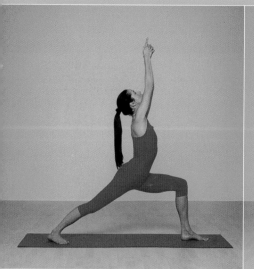

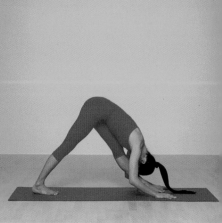

❶ **Warrior** (see pp.40–41)

❷ **Runners' Stretch** (see pp.62–63)

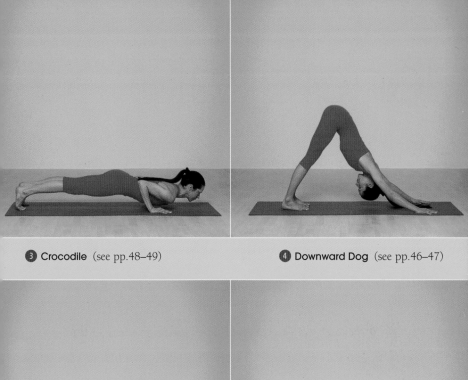

3 Crocodile (see pp.48–49)

4 Downward Dog (see pp.46–47)

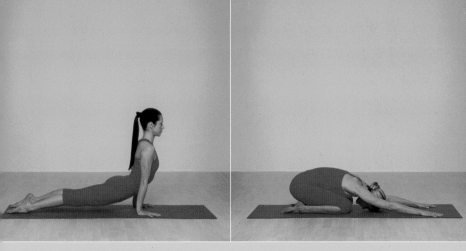

5 Upward Dog (see pp.50–51)

6 Hare (see pp.76–77)

(6) weekend
energizer

Here is an invigorating routine that will set you up for the whole weekend. Integrate the postures with breathe-and-stretch exercises (see p.26), Sun Salute (see p.52), and the Kneeling Stretch sequence (see p.94). Add some breathing practices (see p.100) and the relaxation practice (see p.108) for a longer session.

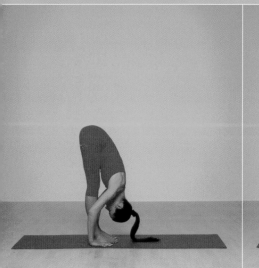

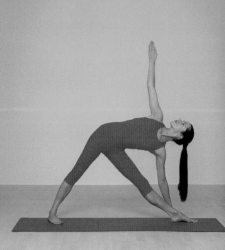

1 Forward Bend (see pp.38–39)   **2** Triangle (see pp.58–59)

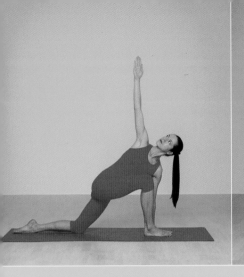

3 Lunge Twist (see pp.64–65)

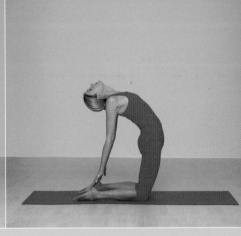

4 Camel (see pp.78–79)

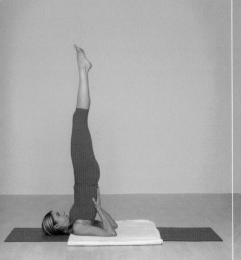

5 Full Shoulder Stand (see pp.84–85)

6 Sitting Forward Stretch (see pp.90–91)

⑦ long journey
reviver

To reduce the stress of long journeys, take frequent breaks during trips to breathe and stretch or to center yourself. At the end of a long journey, the Side-Bending sequence (see p.68), the Kneeling Stretch sequence (see p.94), and the following postures will all help you to unwind. End the program with the relaxation practice (see p.108).

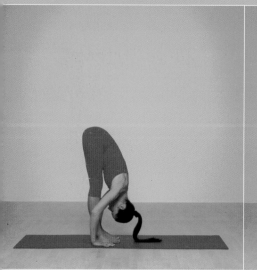

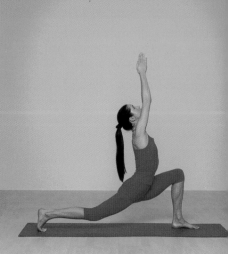

① **Forward Bend** (see pp.38–39)

② **Lunge Warrior** (see pp.42–45)

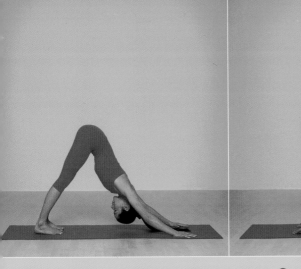

3 Downward Dog (see pp.46–47)

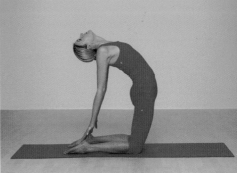

4 Camel (see pp.78–79)

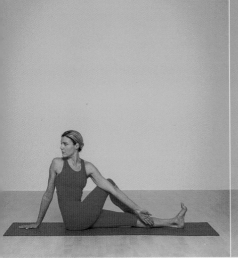

5 Sitting Twist (see pp.98–99)

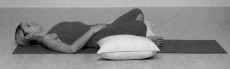

6 Supine Butterfly (see pp.92–93)

Index

Useful organizations

www.yogasite.com
A general source of information on yoga, with good links, and a teachers' directory covering the United States, Canada, Australia, and other countries.

THE BRITISH WHEEL OF YOGA
Tel: 01529 306851;
Website: www.bwy.org.uk
Provides information on classes, yoga organizations, and events in the UK.

www.yogafinder.com
A directory listing yoga teachers, organizations, and events in the United States and other countries.

THE YOGA THERAPY CENTRE
Tel: 020 7869 3040;
Website: www.yogatherapy.org
The Yoga Biomedical Trust's center for yoga therapy, general yoga classes, workshops and training.

Acknowledgments

AUTHOR'S ACKNOWLEDGMENTS
Thanks to my teachers and students, especially Sheri Greenaway, Dr. Shrikrishna and David Swenson; to Julie Bullock and Liz Taylor for help with the text; to Dr. Robin Monro for entrusting me with *Yoga for Living*; to Jane and Anne-Marie for their tireless editorial and design work and for being such fun to work with, and to Nicky and Schroeder for surviving the past year.

PUBLISHER'S ACKNOWLEDGMENTS
Thanks to Catherine MacKenzie for design assistance; Helen Ridge, Jane Simmonds, and Angela Wilkes for editorial assistance; Dorothy Frame for indexing; Katy Wall for jacket design; and Anna Bedewell for additional picture research.

Models: Jean Hall, Lee Hamblin, Cate Williams **Photographer's Assistant:** Nick Rayment **Hair and Makeup:** Hitoko Honbu (represented by Hers)
Studio: Air Studios Ltd

Yoga mats: Hugger Mugger Yoga Products, 12 Roseneath Place, Edinburgh EH9 1JB. **Tel**: 44 (0) 131 221 9977; **Fax**: 44 (0) 131 2291 9112; **Website**: www.yoga.co.uk; **email**: info @huggermugger.co.uk
In the US, these mats can be obtained from: Hugger Mugger Products, 3937 SO 500 W, Salt Lake City, Utah 84123. **Tel**: 800 473 4888; **Fax**: 801 268 2629; **Website**: www.huggermugger.com
Yoga props: Yoga Matters, 42 Priory Road, London N8 7EX. **Tel**: 44 (0) 20 8348 1203; **Website**: www.yogamatters.co.uk; **email**: enquiries@yogamatters.co.uk

PICTURE CREDITS
The publisher would like to thank the following for their kind permission to reproduce their photographs.
7: Getty Images/Pete Turner;
12: Getty Images /Jaques Copean
All other images © Dorling Kindersley. For further information see: www.dkimages.com